The Anatomy of Medical Error

PREVENTING HARM WITH PEOPLE-BASED PATIENT SAFETY™

by E. Scott Geller, Ph.D.
and Dave Johnson

Published by

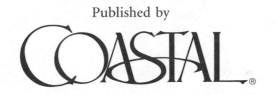

Dedicated to the university students
and our colleagues who collected and analyzed the data
to make this book evidence-based;
to the Partners of Safety Performance Solutions
who help organizations worldwide execute the principles
of People-Based Patient Safety™;
and to the sales personnel of Coastal Training
Technologies Corp. who help people realize the value
of the information presented in this book,
supplementary materials and relevant consulting services.

Published by
Coastal Training Technologies Corporation
500 Studio Drive, Virginia Beach, Virginia 23452
757-498-9014 • www.coastal.com

Library of Congress Control Number Provided Upon Request
ISBN 0-9664604-1-3

Printed in the United States of America

Contents

Preface

All humans — including the most conscientious, highly trained professionals — unintentionally act in ways that can cause harm. It's the nature of human error. Humans are fallible — and human error is often predicable and controllable. The real question is how can we catch these errors before patients are harmed. The purpose of the book in your hands, *The Anatomy of Medical Error*, is to provide you with answers.

Eliminating human error begins with a deeper understanding of human nature, including why we make mistakes and take calculated risks. When we understand the "why's" and learn how to stop ourselves before we do things that could cause unintentional injury, we can act to prevent harm. That's what People-Based Patient Safety™ is all about.

So how do you stop people from taking calculated risks and intentionally or unintentionally making errors that put people at risk?

In the following pages you'll learn how to apply ACTS — Acting, Coaching, Thinking and Seeing — specific skills you can gain and actions you can take to prevent human error.

We start with Acting because our actions — our behavior — is the common denominator. When we understand human behavior and why we do what we do, we can pinpoint critical actions and safety checks before we act. Then we can make the right choices and act to prevent errors.

Coaching is the second component of People-Based Patient Safety™. We know the healthcare system contributes to medical errors, but what is a system? It's an interdependent group of people with a common mission. People — every one of us — are the critical link that makes a system work. When we work interdependently, we save lives. It takes specific skills and that's what Coaching is all about.

In Coaching, we show you the five critical steps to team-oriented healthcare — COACH — Care, Observe, Analyze, Communicate and Help.

Beyond working together to build safety cultures, people have a need to understand why, to interpret their daily experiences and make sense of their lives and relationships. We do this by thinking or through self-talk — that little voice, or monologue in our head. Thinking is the third element of People-Based Patient Safety™.

Errors can happen in a split second when we're distracted, or we stop paying attention to the task at hand. We let our guard down. We bypass mindful self-talk and put ourselves on automatic pilot. Often it happens when we've done a task correctly so many times, it becomes routine.

Mindfulness protects us from the consequences of automatic thinking — and forgetfulness. Before every task, we pause for a few seconds and return to the present moment. We're fully present, observing what is actually before us. We're mindful — we're thinking about the task at hand.

In the chapter on Thinking, we show you how to prompt yourself to think about safety with a mental checklist to stay mindfully focused. To prompt yourself to ask, What am I thinking now? We also show you how to use mental imagery to picture each step you need to take with a questioning mindset; to think about your course of action and be mindful of what is needed to prevent harm to yourself or others.

The fourth part of ACTS is Seeing. When our eyes (and our perceptions) play tricks on us, patients are put at risk. We need to spot the hazards before it's too late. In the chapter on Seeing, we show you how a combination of factors — the limitations of the human eye, our thinking process, even our attitudes and beliefs — can distort perception so we don't see what's right in front of us. Or we see something that isn't actually there.

We present a simple environmental assessment process to help you see the hazards and risks that are often missed — and deal with each one step by step, so we're always aware of what we're doing at all times. Then we show you how we can train ourselves to be more observant of potential behavioral risks and environmental factors that can lead to error. We keep alternating strategically between focusing and scanning throughout the day. We do this to spot hazards and potential errors before it's too late.

Beyond the specifics of ACTS, the heart of People-Based Patient Safety™ is the need for us to view each other as people — rather than objects, titles, job classifications, or a means to an end. People-Based Patient Safety™ requires a very sincere, honest appreciation of other people. It requires an understanding and acceptance of the internal feelings, needs and perceptions of everyone in the organizational culture. Each person's uniqueness and individuality must be recognized.

In the following pages you'll read numerous case studies from the frontlines and interviews with patient-safety experts that demonstrate how this human side of healthcare is improving patient safety, quality of care, and building the organizational safety cultures needed to reduce unintended error and harm.

Use *The Anatomy of Medical Error*, its tools, ideas and frontline accounts, to improve communication, teamwork, as well as interpersonal relationships with your patients and your peers. This is the people side of patient safety.

Acknowledgments

People-Based Patient Safety™ includes the psychological principles and procedures most relevant to patient safety that have been addressed in ten industrial safety books I've authored over the last decade. Thus, the content in this book has benefited from the cumulative advice, support and inspiration of literally hundreds of colleagues, teachers, students and safety leaders. My prior books thanked many of these individuals. For this Acknowledgment, I recognize those with whom I worked directly to accomplish my part of this scholarship.

First, and foremost, I'm grateful for the talent, dedication and insight of my coauthor, Dave Johnson, whose skilled interviewing of numerous healthcare personnel, including physicians, nurses and hospital administrators, informed the selection and revision of the research-based information for this book. Specific dialogue from many of these interviews is reported in this book as testimony to the relevance or value of the information we provide.

As a friend and professional colleague for almost 20 years, Dave has taught me how to translate academic theory and research into real-world language for public service. Dave was the editor of three of my occupational safety books, and each of those books benefited greatly from his expert journalism. But none of that can compare to the meritorious dedication and talent Dave has contributed to this collaborative effort. I am extremely proud to be his coauthor.

Each part of this book is based on an article published in my "Psychology of Safety" column in *Industrial Safety and Hygiene News* (*ISHN*), which Dave Johnson edits. To date, I've authored 173 articles for *ISHN*, and the best 72 of these are included here and supplemented with healthcare information and interviews obtained by my coauthor. Our delivery of information is made more interesting and instructive by illustrations drawn by George Wills, an extremely talented artist who has helped me add humor to my books and keynote addresses for almost two decades.

Since the first drafts of my scholarship are handwritten, I am always indebted to someone's word-processing skills. For this book, I had the very best. Matt Cox and Kristin Williamson coordinated the challenge of preparing the text and illustrations for the publisher. I am profoundly grateful for the special commitment and care these colleagues gave to People-Based Patient Safety™.

Finally, I sincerely appreciate the dedication of the talented staff at Coastal Training Technologies Corp. who brought this book to life, beginning with the vision of Bill Anderson who sought a way to address the challenge of improving patient safety with leading-edge principles and procedures of behavioral and cognitive science. Many other Coastal staff made this realization of Bill's dream possible, including the healthcare advice and editing of Deborah Seymour Taylor, Denise Miller, Anita Brennan, Anne Lewis and the production skills of Marshall McClure.

But every collaborative achievement benefits from quality leadership, and we all got this from Nancy Kondas. Thank you, Nancy, for inspiring us daily to contribute our specific competencies, interdependently, thereby enabling a synergistic outcome.

I thank you all very much, as well as the hundreds of others who have contributed to my 40 years of preparation to coauthor People-Based Patient Safety™. The synergy from all your sustenance provides a legacy – principles and procedures readers can use to apply human dynamics to the prevention of human error in hospitals and other medical facilities, thereby improving patient safety and the quality of healthcare.

E. Scott Geller
August, 2006

In early October 2005 I emailed Ilene Corina, founder of PULSE, a patient-safety advocacy group based in Wantagh, New York, explaining that I was "casting my net far and wide" in search of patient-safety experts for a book project. Any effort to acknowledge all those who helped in this project begins with Ilene. Very generous with her time, candid in conveying her knowledge of the field, Ilene indeed opened numerous doors through her many contacts. Ilene's passion, honesty, generosity and dedication turned out to be characteristics I would come across time and again in my interviews.

My reporting benefited from the hard work of many networkers and facilitators in the patient-safety field. Special thanks to Allison "I will make this happen" Sandve of Children's Hospitals and Clinics of Minnesota; communications consultant Naida Grunden; Linda Zespy with the Safest in America healthcare systems alliance in Minnesota; Vince Rivard of Regions Hospital in St. Paul, Minnesota; Dale Gauding with Sentara Healthcare, Norfolk, Virginia; and Jennifer Amundson with Fairview Health Services, Minneapolis, Minnesota.

Reporters can't report without understanding the broader context of their subject, and essential background information was generously provided by Joe McFadden of McFadden Associates; Martin Hatlie, J.D., president, Partnership for Patient Safety; Charles Inlander, People's Medical Society; Mark Graber, M.D.; Edward F. Minoque, M.D., director, Maryland Patient Safety Center; Raymond Catton, M.D.; James Naughton, M.D.; Denise Miller, RN; Rosemary Gibson, author of *Wall of Silence*; and risk communication consultant Peter Sandman, Ph.D.

Excellent resources I tapped into throughout this project recommended to anyone researching the patient-safety field are the Agency for Healthcare Research & Quality's *Morbidity & Mortality Rounds* on the Web and the National Patient

Safety Foundation list-serv. And anyone's required reading list should include *To Do No Harm* by Julianne Morath and Joanne Turnbull; Rosemary Gibson's *Wall of Silence*; *Complications* by Atul Gawande, M.D.; *Critical Condition* by Donald Barlett and James Steele; *Internal Bleeding* by Robert Wachter, M.D., and Kaveh G. Shojania, M.D.; Florence Nightingale's seminal *Notes on Nursing*; and any interview with or article by Jeffrey Cooper, Ph.D.; David W. Bates, M.D.; Lucian Leape, M.D.; and Donald Berwick, M.D.

Any book project is a collaborative effort, and thanks go to the publishing team at Coastal Training Technologies — Anne Lewis, Bill Anderson and Nancy Kondas — for their encouragement, feedback, ideas and support. Special thanks to Nancy Kondas for being the catalyst and project leader. Of course, Dr. E. Scott Geller is the biggest contributor to the project and the team. His more than 30 years of research in behavioral safety are indispensable to this book's content. Scott's passion to "make a difference," his optimism and energy, and his openness to new ideas make for a very close, comfortable writing partnership. Thanks, partner.

Speaking of partners, I'm grateful to my wife, Suze, for her coaching and superior emotional intelligence in dealing with a writer on deadline. And to my kids, Kate and Steve, for knowing when best to leave Dad alone with his writing.

Dave Johnson
August, 2006

CHAPTER 1 *Getting Going*

In this chapter you'll learn:

1 Prerequisites for patient-safety improvement
Building blocks for a Patient-Safety Culture

Prerequisite: REVOLUTIONARY THINKING

As you would expect, the level of commitment to patient safety is all over the board across the 7,569 hospitals in the United States:[1]

• Some healthcare systems are justly proud of patient-safety activities that predate the Institute of Medicine's (IOM) landmark 1999 report, *To Err is Human*,[2] which opened the nation's eyes to an estimated 44,000 to 98,000 patient deaths each year due to medical errors, and presaged the current patient-safety movement.

• Many healthcare cultures are preoccupied with meeting the annual national patient safety goals and requirements published by the Joint Commission on Accreditation of Healthcare Organizations (JCAHO).

• Some give patient safety more lip service than resources.

• And some raise the bar above the minimums established by accreditation requirements. Impressively, as of this writing, more than 3,000 hospitals have committed to the Institute for Healthcare Improvement's 100,000 Lives Campaign, which targets six patient-safety measures that could save as many as 100,000 lives if even 2,000 hospitals adopted them.[3]

Most American hospitals are safe for the majority of patients most of the time, state the authors of *Internal Bleeding*, describing the vast majority of care-givers as well trained and conscientious.[4] But clearly, many healthcare systems are in the embryonic phase of formally addressing patient safety.

In one study, 92 percent of surveyed hospitals did not have a budget line item for patient safety, and many struggled to define just what constitutes a patient-safety activity.[5] Others wrestle to define the roles, responsibilities and compensation packages for patient-safety officers. The majority of physicians in one poll believed the IOM's estimate of errors and deaths was too high, others dispute proposed solutions.[6]

"Much of what we see in the works these days is simply a rehash of what went before," wrote an observer on the National Patient Safety Foundation's list-serv.[7] Too much talk, not enough action, was his bottom line.

Speaking of finances, the majority of hospitals have invested relatively modest resources in patient-safety activities.[8]

So where are we? You might debate the IOM's estimates, but there's no questioning the unprecedented magnitude of discussion surrounding medical errors and patient-safety issues. Books, articles, research, conferences, workshops, associations, goals, requirements and recommendations propel the patient-safety movement, triggering debates, soul searching and head scratching. Varying degrees of commitment and innovation can be found, along with evidence of institutional inertia.

Where are we? In the midst of a lot of churning. So how do we turn the storming and forming into constructive action?

The starting point: "I receive many calls from people asking where they should start with patient safety," says Julianne M. Morath, M.S., R.N., the chief operating officer and chief nurse executive for Children's Hospitals and Clinics of Minnesota. "We need a thought revolution. The veil of secrecy surrounding errors and harm is just now being lifted."

Drawing on our experience (more than 50 years total) with safety cultures in high-risk industries, we'll jump-start this analysis of medical error and the strategies to prevent patient harm by defining revolutionary thinking, in terms of patient safety. Here are ten principles to frame this new way of thinking — and to energize and sustain a Patient-Safety Culture.

1) From compliance to ownership and commitment

With its primary focus on interpreting externally derived patient-safety requirements, such as the Joint Commission on Accreditation of Healthcare Organization's (JCAHO) policies, the healthcare industry reminds us of general industry's attitude that equates worker safety with whatever the Occupational Safety and Health Administration (OSHA) declares must be done.

Since OSHA's creation within the Department of Labor in 1970, most safety investments by general industry have been driven by federal rules. In a 2004 survey, 74 percent of companies with more than 1,000 employees reported OSHA compliance as the main factor behind safety investments; in contrast, 52 percent pointed to cultural values of employee protection.[9] Four of the top five worker-safety training topics related specifically to OSHA requirements in a 2002 survey of workplaces.[10]

In other words, many organizations in industry "do safety" because the government requires it, which has a stifling effect on research and innovation. People in any line of work will be more motivated and willing to go beyond the call of duty when they perceive they are achieving their own self-initiated goals, rather than when they are merely fulfilling requirements set by someone else.

OSHA doesn't "own" workplace safety anymore than JCAHO "owns" patient safety. Ownership is an inside job — grown organically from within organizations.

2) From failure-avoidance to success-seeking

When people work to fulfill someone else's requirements rather than to achieve their own goals, they are apt to develop an attitude of "working to avoid failure" rather than "working to achieve success." Scoring systems fixated on failure facilitate this negative orientation. In terms of patient safety, this might mean medication errors, sentinel events, infection rates, etc.

People feel more in control when working to achieve than when working to avoid failure. They display more consistent attention, less procrastination, and a healthier attitude when working to achieve quality healthcare and patient-safety goals than when working to avoid blame, punishment or embarrassment.

Giving patient safety an achievement perspective requires a different scoring system, as applied in the next new perspective.

3) From outcome-focused to behavior-focused

Here we are not referring to outcomes of medical procedures and treatment, but rather results of patient-safety activities. We have concerns, for example, about the proliferation of ranking systems to grade the performance of hospitals using patient-safety criteria.

We've learned from general industry that providing incentives for lower numbers (such as sentinel events, patient falls, and medication errors) can often reduce the numbers (that is, the reported outcomes) while not improving safety.

When attention goes to reducing outcomes without changing the process (such as ongoing safety-related behaviors), employees often cover up their mistakes. This keeps outcome numbers low, but does more harm than good to the overall culture of safety.

A scoring system based on what people do for safety (a behavior-based process) not only attacks the root causes of most errors and failures, but can also be achievement-oriented. This places patient safety in the same motivational framework as quality medical

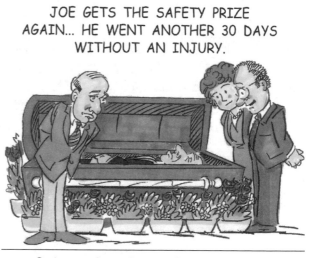

JOE GETS THE SAFETY PRIZE AGAIN... HE WENT ANOTHER 30 DAYS WITHOUT AN INJURY.

Outcome-based rewards remove focus from action.

diagnosis and treatment. (We fully explain the behavior-based approach in Chapter 2 on Acting.)

4) From top-down control to bottom-up involvement

A behavior-based, achievement focus on patient safety requires continual involvement from frontline caregivers. They have the front-row seats to spot where risks are greatest and when at-risk behaviors occur.

Also, caregivers — by their very name — have the most influence in supporting safe, caring behaviors and correcting at-risk behaviors (and conditions).

In fact, ongoing processes involved in developing a Patient-Safety Culture need to be supported from the top but driven from the bottom. This is more than employee participation; it is employee ownership, commitment and empowerment.

5) *From rugged individualism to teamwork*

A patient-safety process that grows organically within units and departments requires teamwork founded on trust. But from childhood most of us have been taught an individualistic, win/lose perspective, supported by such pop mantras as "Looking out for Number One," "He with the most toys wins," and "Nice guys finish last."

That tradition carries over into medicine, which risk communication expert Peter Sandman calls "radically individualistic…with every doctor a rugged individualist."

To be sure, a true team approach to patient safety involving, among other tactics, interpersonal observation and feedback of safe versus at-risk work practices is not easy to pull off. It runs counter to healthcare's ingrained culture of autonomy, fiefdoms, and decentralized decision-making.

"Collaboration is built through conversation, information, and shared purpose in work," says Morath, coauthor of the book, *To Do No Harm*, published in 2005. "Over a nice dinner we asked doctors and nurses how we could make our hospital care safer. They talked about teamwork and communication, a more reliable process to communicate and work together. Then a light bulb turned on. We can use teams! We can make transfer points less vulnerable. It became very apparent to physicians that their exposure to risk would be reduced by having another set of eyes watching and information being shared."

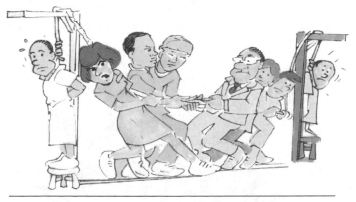

Some cultures promote win/lose independency over win/win interdependency.

6) *From a piecemeal perspective to a systems approach*

A true Patient-Safety Culture can only be achieved with a systems approach. Whenever you obtain a list of factors contributing to a patient-safety incident or near hit, categorize them into three areas (which we call the Safety Triad):

I. environmental factors (such as equipment, availability and access to supplies, signage, labeling, how work is staffed and organized, housekeeping, temperature control, lighting);

II. personal factors (employees' knowledge, skills, abilities, intelligence, motives, personality);

III. behavioral factors (employees complying, recognizing, communicating, "actively caring").

Two of these categories involve human factors. Each of these generally receives less attention than the environment, largely because it's more difficult to document outcomes of efforts to influence human factors.

The most common reaction to an error that harmed or could have harmed a patient is to correct something in the environment (alarms, equipment operation, communication systems, recordkeeping systems, housekeeping, lighting, temperature control, bed railings, etc.).

Often an incident report includes some mention of person factors (the employee's knowledge, skills, ability, intelligence, motives, or personality), but these factors are typically translated into general corrective action recommendations like: "The employee will be disciplined" or "the employee will be retrained."

This lack of penetrating analysis to the critical human component of a patient-safety incident reflects frustration in dealing with person factors. But the human aspect of an incident can be addressed through behavior. Indeed, the person factors can be influenced by careful attention to behaviors, environments, and the fact there can be pleasant consequences to unsafe behavior (or unpleasant consequences to safe behavior). More on this in Chapter 2 on Acting.

Some human factors programs focus on behavior-based safety management; others focus on attitudes (as in a person-based approach). An authentic Patient-Safety Culture requires integrating both behavior-based and person-based approaches in order to understand and influence human dynamics within an organizational culture. We call this People-Based Patient Safety™.[11]

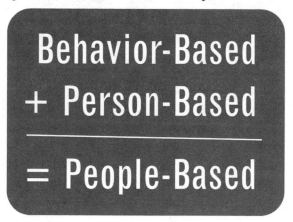

7) From fault-finding to fact-finding

Blaming a particular individual or group of individuals for an error or failure is not consistent with a systems approach to safety.

Instead, unintended harm to a patient or a near hit[12] provides an opportunity to analyze facts from all aspects of the system that could have contributed to the incident. Not only are the immediate environment, person, and behavior factors explored as potential contributors, but numerous historical factors can be considered.

How common, for example, was the at-risk behavior? How many people observed the at-risk behavior without intervening? And what aspects of operations and the management system supported the at-risk behavior?

8) *From reactive to proactive*

Investigating circumstances preceding an incident reveals the need to think and act proactively. Unfortunately, a proactive posture is a strain to maintain, especially in healthcare systems where hours worked, patients per caregiver, available medications, procedures and practice specialties are all increasing, resulting in a higher price tag on "free time."

With barely enough time to react effectively and safely to the crises of the day, how can we find time to be proactive?

9) *From quick fix to continuous improvement*

Obviously there is no quick-fix answer. Only with a systems perspective and an optimistic mindset of continuous improvement can "proactive" replace "reactive."

10) *From priority to value*

As long as patient safety is a priority, it is legitimate to shift its priority ranking depending on other priorities at the time. It usually takes external forces (such as JCAHO goals and various accreditation requirements, media reporting, federal or state legislation, CEO turnover) to boost the priority ranking of patient safety.

When individuals and an organizational culture hold patient safety as a value, however, there is no compromise for safety. The "safe way" is embedded within each of the priorities of the day, no matter how quickly they might change.

Each of the ten revolutionary shifts discussed here should be considered a "transition mission" to complete in order to achieve a Patient-Safety Culture. That is, patient-safety processes should be seen as both organizational and individual responsibilities. Your Patient-Safety Culture must be achievement-oriented, with a focus on behaviors, and developed organically through coaching and teamwork.

A systems approach is necessary, which leads to a fact-finding perspective, a proactive stance, and an appreciation of continuous improvement. With these perspectives, it is indeed possible to shift patient safety from a current priority to a lasting, embedded value.

Prerequisite: FEELINGS

Many professional people, especially those with backgrounds in science or engineering — the "hard stuff" — view psychology as a subjective "touchy-feely" discipline. But psychological principles are founded on objective empirical research, not on common sense.

So along with the sciences of engineering and medicine, we have the science of human behavior. Just as we have engineering and medical technology to benefit our quality of life, we also have behavioral technology to improve human performance.

That said, there is a "soft" side to psychology. Consider this fundamental principle of human nature: We all react to the way others feel about us. When we sense management or another unit or another shift doesn't really care about what we're doing, patient-safety processes requiring collaboration and interdependence will fail.

It's a formidable challenge to make collaboration acceptable in a decentralized, results-oriented system such as healthcare. But without a people-focused, collaborative mindset, system performance will always be less than optimal — whether it's measured in terms of error reduction and patient-safety injuries or quality, customer service or productivity.

We are similarly convinced breakthroughs in patient safety will not occur if feelings and emotions are denied. Patient-safety literature is replete with phrases and references that illustrate how feelings and emotions permeate the entire issue: Errors and failures lead to "media lashings" and "emotional fallout" that can leave patients, families and caregivers "devastated," "shattered" and "rocked to the core." A "collective organizational anxiety" and "ongoing unease" can follow. "Compassion," "tenacity," "restored confidence" and "relentless vigilance" are all necessary to calibrate the proper amount of "tension" needed to prevent harm from reaching patients.

Where's the data? But how do you respond to decision-makers demanding data, outcome evidence, to support patient safety interventions? "I run into this all the time," says Jeffrey B. Cooper, Ph.D. Dr. Cooper, a patient-safety pioneer, presented the first in-depth, scientific look at errors in medicine in his 1978 paper, "Preventable Anesthesia Mishaps: A study in human factors," based on an analysis of 359 errors. "We can't wait around for randomized controlled trials while patients are being injured or are dying from preventable causes. You've got to do some things that reasonable people agree on," Dr. Cooper says.

Today he says, "Industry is more willing to accept and work with much less tangible evidence when it comes to safety. Many people in medicine are wired on the left side of the brain and want everything to be measured, to have a suitable "p-value" before acting. But safety is the science of chaotic, rare events that are harder to predict and measure.

"Sometimes I ask, 'Is there nothing you'll buy on face validity?' What's the ROI on a one-hour lecture for clinicians? Some things in medicine are completely driven by anecdotal evidence.

"Healthcare knows its people don't work well in teams, don't communicate well across tribes. 'Where are the data on teamwork?' Well, there is almost no scientific evidence it prevents plane crashes. In more than 50 studies of crisis resource management in aviation, only one mildly established a connection. Still, every airline is doing crew resource management training — with evidence only that it improves performance of the crews in simulators, not that it directly prevents accidents. Do you want to fly an airline that ignores crew resource management?"

Where's the data? "Get off it already," says Dr. Cooper.

Prerequisite: **INTERDEPENDENCE**

We need a global perspective to see the myriad linkages and couplings that bind together a Patient-Safety Culture. This is systems thinking for safety. Here are seven principles that emanate from such a perspective:

1) *There is no single root cause*

Systems thinkers do not try to find one root cause of a close call or harmful incident. At-risk behavior contributes to 95 percent or more of most injuries in general industry workplaces, whether intentional or unintentional.[13] But this does not mean an individual's at-risk behavior is the root cause of the injury. A number of other factors are involved.

2) *Consider environment, behavior and person-based factors*

These factors are interactive, dynamic and reciprocal. An organization's management system is an environmental factor with dramatic impact on human factors. A top-down authoritarian approach might dictate certain compliant behavior, but it also creates a nega-tive attitude that can foster resistance and contrary behaviors. A more open and trusting leadership style will naturally produce a different set of proactive behaviors and attitudes. And a more optimistic and engaged workforce can lead management to open up even further. The spiraling, reciprocal interdependency between the operating environment, behav-iors and person-based factors can influence more behavior change and then more attitude change.

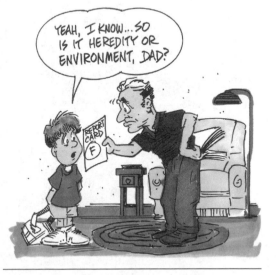

Behavior is influenced by both environment and person factors.

3) *Measure these factors*

Environment and behavior factors can be systematically assessed with periodic audits. Perception and attitude surveys can be useful barometers of person-based factors. Reactive measures of patient safety, such as report cards that tally up mistakes and errors, have absolutely no diagnostic value to help understand or change system variables that contribute to outcomes. Keep in mind that outcome measures are influenced by numerous factors, such as punishment and reward programs that can lead to under-reporting.

4) *Investigate facts, not faults*

This emphasis on facts over faults bears repeating. Systems thinkers (who see error caused by multiple factors, not one individual) attempt to remove any aspect of their environment that could inhibit incident reporting. If factors in the system promote a fault-finding perspective toward error-related investigation, then information critical to preventing errors could be buried. And the fault-finding perspective usually begins with undue focus on outcomes rather than processes.

5) *Feedback directs and motivates*

Systems thinkers don't rush in for the quick fix. They understand cause-and-effect is not necessarily immediate, nor linear. Taking the time to be safe today can help develop a personal routine that pays dividends in the future. Or it could teach others by example and protect patients now or later from injury.

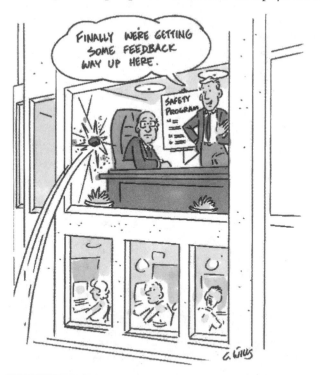

Feedback can be reactive, remote and destructive.

Systems thinkers realize the special need to add extra feedback to activate and motivate safe behavior. They understand the natural feed-back from convenience, comfort, or a faster outcome usually competes with the completely safe way to do something. Why is adherence to hand-hygiene recommendations usually below 50 percent? Access to cleansing materials isn't easy enough, according to one study. [14]

6) *Consistency develops commitment*

When we choose to act in a certain way, we experience internal pressure to maintain a personal belief system or attitude consistent with that behavior. And when we have certain beliefs or attitudes toward something, we tend to behave in ways that are consistent with such beliefs or attitudes. Commitment and involvement result from this synergism.

In your patient-safety activities, leave space for personal choices. When people believe their commitment was their idea, they are more likely to consistently follow through. You've activated the consistency principle. But when people believe their commitment stems from outside requirements or top-down orders, buy-in tends to be superficial. They don't feel a need to "own" someone else's product.[15]

7) *Embrace reciprocity*

Interdependence requires reciprocity. In other words, if you watch someone's back, that person will feel obligated to cover for you. And consistent with a systems perspective, reciprocal acts are not always linear. You help out a teammate, and that teammate can feel motivated to help out another teammate, not necessarily you. Many of the interdependent acts required of a Patient-Safety Culture — everything from lifting patients to verifying prescriptions to incident disclosure and time-outs — benefit from the reciprocity principle.

As you can see from these principles, interdependence changes our perspective from narrowly linear to globally circular. We can see how small changes in behavior can result in attitude change, followed by more behavior change and more desired attitude change, leading eventually to personal commitment and total involvement in a patient-safety process.

Prerequisite: CONVERSATION

Think how seeds of revolution are often sown: patriots bending elbows and brainstorming in Philadelphia and Boston taverns, the founding fathers spending weeks in raucous debates. "We need authentic conversations around patient safety, deeper conversations with disclosure and purpose," says Julianne Morath of the Children's Hospitals and Clinics of Minnesota.

We're talking of the need for two types of conversations. One has to do with our mental scripts — what we say to ourselves (in this case regarding patient-safety issues). The other is our verbal exchanges with others. Powerful beliefs and values are weighed, defined and take root in these conversations. Eventually, the characteristics of a Patient-Safety Culture — whether it is proactive or reactive, fault-finding or fact-finding, based on avoiding failure or seeking success — will be shaped by conversations both spoken and unspoken.

What are the "unspoken conversations" about patient safety in your unit, facility or system — the customs or unwritten rules people heed without mention? Perception surveys are one method to shed light on these hidden norms.

Bottom line: The status of patient safety in your organization is largely determined by how it is talked about. Whether we feel responsible and committed to work toward a breakthrough depends on our interpretation or mental script about these conversations.

It falls to patient-safety coaches, officers, physicians, other frontline personnel, informal leaders and titled executives to set the tone and direction of the conversations that shape your Patient-Safety Culture.

Prerequisite: LANGUAGE

The tone of these conversations will surely be affected by your choice of words. Think how certain expressions actually harm patient-safety efforts.[16]

"Language shapes culture," says Ms. Morath. "Leaders should ask, 'What happened?' instead of 'Who did it?' Replace 'investigations' with 'analytical reviews.' We've eliminated 'incident reports' and replaced them with 'Patient-Safety Learning Reports.'

"There are a lot of emotional connotations — baggage — with the language we've used. It leads to a culture of blame, shame and train."

Here are some other words that should be handled with care, if not eliminated entirely from conversations, if we want to achieve an open and collaborative Patient-Safety Culture.

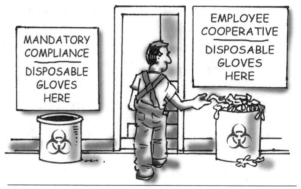

Language affects behavior.

"Accident" implies chance

The first definition of "accident" in the *New Merriam-Webster Dictionary* (copyright 1989) is "an event occurring by chance or unintentionally." In general industry, the idea that "Accidents will happen" can kill motivation to improve safety performance. In healthcare an analogy might be, "Harm happens." We need to stop the shrugging and acceptance of inevitability. Replace it with the belief and expectation that risk can be prevented and patients protected by controlling factors such as environmental conditions, behaviors and attitudes.

Is safety a "priority" or a "value"?

Leaders are often quick to say, "Patient safety should be a priority." This seems appropriate, since the dictionary defines "priority" as "taking precedence logically or in importance." But as we discussed earlier, everyday experience teaches us that priorities come and go. Depending on the demands of the moment, one priority often gets shifted for another. Do we really want to place patient safety on such shifting sands?

In contrast, the relevant definition of "value" in the dictionary is "something (as a principle or ideal) intrinsically valuable or desirable." Patient safety should be a "value" employees bring to every job, regardless of ongoing priorities or task requirements. An organization's mission statement should refer to patient safety as a "value" rather than a "priority."

Here are other word-attitude connotations worth considering:
 • Should we say "peer pressure" or "peer support"?
 • Should we refer to patient-safety leaders as "managers" or "facilitators"?
 • Should we discuss the results of a safety audit as "meeting JCAHO requirements" or "fulfilling an organizational mission"?
 • Do you have a "patient-safety compliance" task force or a "patient-safety achievement" task force?
 • Did a unit go "30 days without an adverse event" or did it work "30 safe days"?

Let's be clear: discussions of patient safety should not be exercises in political correctness. There's already more than enough silvery lip service putting a shine on the subject. Word substitution games can become trivial pursuits. But it can be a useful personal or group exercise to identify the negative connotations associated with various phrases used in patient-safety conversation, and come up with appropriate alternatives in some cases.

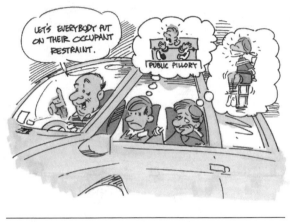

Language can be a turn-off.

Prerequisite: PERSONAL RESPONSIBILITY

We've seen this irony play out in general industry: as organizations develop an infrastructure to support safety activities, the measures taken to pull safety work together under one department, steering committee, or individual, actually create divisions. As in, "Safety? That's not my job. That's what we pay the safety officer to do around here." Or: "Take that up with the safety steering committee."

The same dynamic can undercut patient safety. One person steps to the plate (either as a volunteer or paid specialist) and many employees feel the game's over for them — the responsibility rests with someone else.

"It's not my job." How many times have you heard that? This rationale for "passing the buck" is actually supported by the typical questions we ask when addressing an issue that requires attention, such as patient safety.

Questions that deflect

Questions beginning with "who," "what," and "when" avoid personal responsibility by assigning accountability elsewhere.

"Who dropped the ball on that hand-off?"

"What Red Rule was not followed?"

"When will the company install an adequate computerized physician order entry system?"

These are not bad questions to ask, not at all. They represent the kind of questions needed to identify and solve problems related to patient safety. But they imply the problem — and solution — is beyond the individual. Totally? After all, systems rely on individual contributions to run efficiently and safely.

Surely we can ask "Why?" But be careful. Some "why" questions are nonproductive and facilitate denial of personal responsibility. "Why was I picked to lead the next patient-safety meeting?" "Why me?" These "why" questions activate and support victim thinking and contribute to the avoidance of personal responsibility.

What can I do?

The simple question, "What can I do?" reflects the essence of personal responsibility. A unit analyzes patient-safety incident reports and prioritizes problems that need to be fixed, starting with too many breakdowns in communications. Now is not the time to look back and ask: "Who caused these problems?" or "Why can't they get it together?" or "Whose job is it to fix these misunderstandings?"

Personal responsibility requires looking ahead, not back over your shoulder. "What can I do to help?" That's personal responsibility. Don't ask questions that "pass the buck" to someone else at some later time. Ask, "How can I help?"

But we can't do it all

A caveat: Many patient-safety issues have no simple solution. A long-term investment of financial and interpersonal resources is needed. As a result, it's easy to deny personal responsibility with the claim, "There's nothing I can do without more support."

The systems picture can seem overwhelming, and systems solutions can seem remote even with substantial support. But doing nothing improves nothing, and could risk more errors and patient harm. So break it down. Find something small within your own domain of influence that relates to the problem and take personal responsibility to perform that action.

Start by defining the problem in terms of actions or behaviors, then identify talents or work assignments related to each action, and then select something from this list you can accomplish. Personal responsibility starts by creating this list of problem-related activities. Consider persuading someone else to take on a solution-related assignment commensurate with his or her talent and position in the organization. Then find others to contribute within their domain of personal control.

Expert Q&A *"I don't ever want to tell another family this again."*

David Page is president and chief executive officer of Fairview Health Services, Minneapolis, Minnesota, and chair of Safest in America, a coalition of 10 healthcare systems and 27 hospitals in the Minneapolis-St. Paul area plus the Mayo Clinic in Rochester, Minnesota.

Q *How did you come to possess a deep-seated conviction in the importance of reducing medical errors?*

A *I have some vivid memories. Some years ago, when I was with another organization, I was attending a conference in Atlanta. I got a call in my hotel room at six-thirty in the evening. We had just had a wrongful death, a medical mishap. An infant under the age of two had died as a result of a massive medical error.*

I thought, "My God, what was going on?" and I caught a plane back home late that night. We had a team discussion in my office at seven the next morning. It was not a particularly productive meeting. We didn't conduct a root-cause analysis or anything like that. We met again in the afternoon. My contribution to these meetings was minimal. But my flying back from the conference helped the organization absorb the seriousness of a case like this.

I remember once telling a husband that his wife, who was in for outpatient treatment, was in mortal danger in the ICU due to a respiratory event. She never came home to her children. Doctors may go through this a lot, but I haven't. It left a strong memory and made a strong impression on me.

I didn't think, "These things happen." I thought, "My God, this is horrible. I don't ever want to tell another family this again."

As a senior leader, your lowest moments come when you have doubts — "Are we really this bad?" It's the worst thing to get these calls or have these conversations.

I was in my early 50s when it became clear to me that healthcare is inherently dangerous, and I came out of the closet. I'm a convert, a zealot about patient safety.

Prerequisite: ACTION

We're talking about going into action, however narrow in scope that may be initially. Yes, seeds of a Patient-Safety Culture are sown in conversations, and take more defined shape through brainstorming, planning and goal setting. But nothing happens until someone or a group of people acts — an incident is reported, analyzed, and findings shared. Then new procedures are developed and tested. They are observed and modified as needed, and measured to test for improvements. Accomplishments are to be celebrated, even in subtle acts of recognition.

Now let's consider four mental barriers that impede action:

"That's the way it is."

In cultures where the behavior of people in leadership positions is not consistent with patient-safety rules and regulations, the stage is set for compromising safety in the name of efficiency. In such a culture, you can expect many opportunities for safety intervention to be overlooked.

"Someone else will help."

The larger the work system, the easier it is to believe someone else will pick up the slack. And in hierarchical systems like healthcare, control is maintained by knowing your place in the pecking order. It's risky to cross the lines of authority. "Let someone else do it."

"What should I do?"

Researchers have shown that individuals are more likely to help others in emergency situations when they know what to do. Observers without relevant training are quick to defer the responsibility to someone else.[17]

Assertiveness training, for example, helps people stand up for their rights and come to the realization their feelings and opinions matter and should be expressed. Such training involves direct instruction and role-playing of specific verbal expressions to regain control in certain situations.[18] Practicing what to say to resolve or alleviate a conflict beforehand enables people to intervene effectively in the "heat" of the moment. Likewise, practicing what to say before asking a peer to work safely will increase the likelihood you'll actually intervene and be effective. Instead of saying, "Why don't you follow the safe procedure?" ask, "What barriers hold you back from doing as much as possible for patient safety?"

"They got what they deserved."

Have you ever thought that someone, maybe a coworker, who made a mistake did something to deserve it? Social psychologists call this phenomenon the "just world hypothesis" — people assume we get what we deserve and deserve what we get."[19]

Here's hoping the next time you see someone taking a risk relevant to patient safety, you'll overcome these four obstacles and step in for safety's sake.

Ask yourself...

• Have you observed at-risk behavior and said to yourself, "What a careless thing to do; if he gets caught, he deserves to be punished"?

• Have you avoided getting involved in a situation because you felt untrained or ill-equipped to deal with it?

• Have you ever held back from speaking up for patient safety because you figured someone else would or should help?

• Have you held back because you felt your work environment condoned risky behavior?

Expert Q&A *"Getting it"*

Jeffrey B. Cooper, PhD, is a patient-safety pioneer. His 1978 paper, "Preventable Anesthesia Mishaps: A Study in Human Factors," was the first in-depth, scientific look at errors in medicine, based on analysis of 359 errors. Today, Dr. Cooper is director of biomedical engineering for Partners HealthCare System, Inc.; associate professor of anesthesia at Harvard Medical School; and executive director of the Center for Medical Simulation in Cambridge, Massachusetts.

Q *You've stated a lot of people still don't "get it" regarding patient safety. Define "getting it." What are the indicators, the behaviors, of someone who "gets it" or a culture that "gets it"?*

A *An organization gets it when people openly discuss and share stories of errors. They don't feel they have to keep it inside.*

Several years ago we had a significant event, a potentially devastating failure relating to how a nurse used a device that had a software bug after it had been upgraded. We pulled people together like in the Apollo 13 crisis and solved the problem. I said our story should be in The Wall Street Journal. *The response I got was something like, "You've got to be kidding!" When I say, "They didn't get it," I mean they didn't see the value in publicizing a near failure that was really a success and a learning experience for others. You must be willing to look vulnerable or weak and risk reporting your story.*

I look for signs of small cultural shifts. Once a technician who worked in our department came into my office and told me about a mistake he made that almost caused a serious injury. I thanked him for telling me and told him how important it was that he was honest when he could have easily hidden it. He felt he was just doing his job. At the time I was working on a patient-safety recognition program for my department, but he didn't want an award. He got the first award anyway.

Another time there was a meeting where significant event cases were being presented for review. During a presentation, a first-year resident stood up and said, "This is my case." Someone else was making the presentation. He didn't have to do that. The fact that he did said to me the culture was starting to change.

2 Ten strategies to get you going

Tap into knowledge of the problem and compassion for patients

Start talking.

The old mental model of risk went something like this: if a mistake happens, file a report, put it away, and hope no one ever asks about it, a nurse told us. "How screwed up is that?" she exclaimed. "Or," she continued, "if harm to a patient did happen, we'd finger ourselves for blame and be silenced by shame."

Healthcare is deeply rooted in altruism, she continued. "We all want to help people. And we know you can do everything right and still harm someone." If you're looking for a starting place to build momentum for patient safety, start talking in a way that addresses what's in the head of your caregivers — their knowledge of the problems — and in their hearts — sincere compassion for patients.

Get your mandate.

The old mantra from industry — "Safety starts at the top" — applies to any work culture. Talk about patient-safety issues all you want, but to turn conversations into interventions you must "get clear mandates from your leadership," says Peter Perreiah, managing director of the Pittsburgh Regional Healthcare Initiative.

Here's one example: "We require direct conversations with patients about errors," says Brock Nelson, president and chief executive officer of Regions Hospital in St. Paul, Minnesota. "We expect these conversations to be held."

There's another saying from industry: "Don't give me management's support, give me their involvement."

You see, "support" can be passive. Management support for patient safety can be as simple as decreeing policies and mission statements. A Patient-Safety Culture requires energy beyond edicts. There is a "direct dose-response relationship" between senior executive involvement and patient-safety attitude survey scores, notes Lori Paine, patient-safety coordinator for The Johns Hopkins Hospital. The more frequently executives work with teams, the higher the scores are from that team on the Safety Attitude Questionnaire.

Set your sights.

"There is a tangled web of patient-safety problems resulting from old, broken systems," says Paine. "It can be quite overwhelming." Some systems have been broken for so long, with Band-Aid on top of Band-Aid, how do you break through the sense of helplessness?

Take the time to study incident reports, collect other sources of data, and analyze the roots of problems. You'll find the low-hanging fruit, says Paine. It's important to find early wins with patient safety.

Another option is a simple survey tool used at Hopkins. Staff is asked: Where is the next patient in this unit going to be harmed? What can we do to prevent that harm?

"Allow frontline people to express their concerns," concludes Paine.

Define roles and responsibilities.

Set your sights, find your targets, develop an action plan – that's all well and good, but execution requires accountability. And in many cultures where patient safety still lacks formal support structures, erecting an accountability system can be difficult. Unfortunately, you won't succeed without one.

For example, The Johns Hopkins Hospital challenges patient-safety teams to find and fix one defect a month – problems identified through its reporting system. At the Children's Hospitals and Clinics of Minnesota, teams are accountable for identifying and coming up with a solution for one patient-safety-related project each year.

Feed organic growth.

Once you give direction and point the way, as a patient-safety coach or coordinator, you need to step back and allow a project team room to breathe. "We strive for organic growth of teams," says Paine. Leadership within the team must champion the project, she says. Coaches provide advice and facilitate disputes, but getting team members to accept personal responsibility comes from within. Don't smother your team with advice.

Track performance.

Designed during your planning stages, metrics will be the rails laid down in advance to prevent teams and projects from skidding off track. Rigorous pre- and post-intervention data assessments are a key component of team activity at The Johns Hopkins Hospital. And teams should monitor and measure interventions while in progress. Without ongoing measurement, there's no sense of momentum or progress.

Celebrate early and often.

If you've given a team a year to work on a patient-safety goal, don't wait 365 days to recognize their time and effort. "Celebrate early milestones," says one patient-safety leader. By recognizing and applauding process activities along the way and not just ultimate outcomes, you allow your teams to "re-fuel" for the long haul.

Pace yourself.

It's a long journey indeed. Just look at the strategies we've outlined. "Authentic," open and probing conversations to get things going consume time and mental energy. Securing not just leadership support but active participation challenges the best sales and diplomacy skills. Collecting data, assessing risks, setting goals, drawing up action plans, designing metrics, assigning roles and responsibilities — it's all intense detail work beyond the already busy schedule of healthcare professionals.

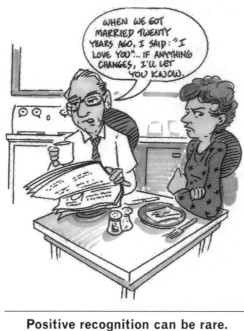

Positive recognition can be rare.

To which we say: 1) Pace yourself and 2) Don't go it alone.

Find allies to help you sell, market and communicate; and watch for signs of burn-out – both in yourself and in your teams. We've seen too many safety professionals in industry pride themselves on being lone rangers, the only ones who can come in, clean up and fix a safety mess. Here's another irony we've noticed: It requires passion and confidence to tackle an organizational issue like safety, which is often given short shrift. But too much passion and confidence distances and alienates safety advocates from the rest of the organization. They become isolated, and unable to accomplish the very thing they set out to do.

3 Common cultural barriers
The paralyzing effects of fear, fatalism, fatigue, fog and frustration

In our interviews for this book, patient-safety experts pointed to numerous obstacles to preventing medical errors. The list is lengthy and disconcerting, so we edited it down to five factors that can paralyze organizations:

Fear
    Fear of blame. Punishment. Malpractice. Loss of credentials. Loss of autonomy. Alarming the public. Losing out to competition. Alienating peers. Intimidation. Bullying. Getting your lunch eaten. All possible negatives for stepping out and speaking up for patient safety, for refusing to pass the buck.
    W. Edwards Deming implored leaders to drive fear out of organizations. That campaign must start at the top.[20]
    "There is never any punishment or blame if it turns out a stoppage was not necessary," says Julianne Morath. "People are thanked for doing it, regardless. We never diminish the action in service of creating greater safety and protecting a patient from potential harm."

Fatalism

Broken systems promote fatalism. And many healthcare systems are stressed to the breaking point as excess capacity is squeezed out and infrastructure investments are put off to save money and boost operating margins.[21] At the same time, patient volume has increased. Emergency room visits increased 15 percent from 1988 to 1998 at a time when 1,128 emergency departments closed.[22] Insured patient visits increased 24 percent from 1996 to 2001.[23]

Many caregivers see no way out. "The best people will make mistakes in a crummy system," says one patient-safety expert.

One way out is to deconstruct systems. A growing body of research is studying how to attain short- and long-term peak performance in clinical microsystems. These are small, functional, frontline units that provide the most healthcare to the most people — everything from a family practice to a cardiac surgery team to a neonatal intensive care unit to a home healthcare delivery service.

Many of the prerequisites for patient-safety success we discussed in this chapter have been identified as important building blocks to high-quality microsystem performance, including role alignment, interdependence of teams, ongoing measurement, and support and investment from the larger organization.[24]

Fatigue

Fatigue, of course, can lead to slips, lapses and mistakes, which is one reason why JCAHO proposed as a 2007 national patient-safety goal requiring organizations to identify conditions and practices that contribute to healthcare work fatigue and take action to minimize those risks.[25] We have more to say about the effects of fatigue in Chapter 4 on Thinking.

Fog

"Not many healthcare institutions have a good sense of where they are — good, bad or average — with patient safety," one nurse told us. But don't use missing benchmarks, metrics, and validated outcome data as excuses for doing nothing, she stressed, adding, "What if it's your mother in the operating room?"

To try to peer through the fog, a growing number of healthcare systems use culture perception surveys to get a reading on current patient-safety attitudes and opinions. Robust reporting systems, which lead first to root-cause analyses and then on to networks that disseminate lessons learned, also help disperse the fog. Perception surveys are discussed in more detail in Chapter 5 on Seeing.

Frustration

The litany of frustrations in healthcare is as daunting as a list of fears. Waste and inefficiencies, patient flows beyond any one individual's control, piles of paperwork, remote and preoccupied leadership, maintenance delays, scheduling interruptions and bureaucratic annoyances — all are sources of ire.

These frustrations lead to many of the at-risk behaviors we discuss in Chapter 2 on Acting; lapses in critical thinking we take up in Chapter 4 on Thinking; and the perceptual biases we explain in Chapter 5 on Seeing.

4 Patient-safety myths
How to respond to typical biases

Be prepared to confront these perceptual (and perpetual) biases as you work to embed patient-safety values in your organization:

"It won't happen here."
Many medical errors occur in relative isolation, in one corner of a very complex system. Incident story-telling involving caregivers and patients and root-cause analyses findings are ways of communicating and reminding staff that yes, incidents and close calls are always happening somewhere in the system.

"Only careless people cause errors."
It is critical to distinguish between intentional versus unintentional neglect because this difference determines the nature of the intervention or corrective action to stop such neglect. If neglect is unintentional, education and training can work. But if neglect is intentional, contingencies or consequences are needed. This might involve incentives, disincentives, or corrective coaching.

"These things happen."
A mindset of inevitability is tantamount to learned helplessness or failure acceptance. Shrugging off errors is clearly detrimental to patient welfare and failure acceptance causes distress to caregivers. We experience stress (beneficial motivation) when we are in control, but experience distress (debilitating motivation) when the perception of control is absent. It's essential to focus on feasible interventions to improve patient safety. This relates to the notion of seeking success rather than avoiding failure.

"I'm doing all I can."
Again, it's important to assess intent. We expect healthcare workers to be well intentioned, meaning they want to do their best to reduce errors that can harm patients. These intentions need only education and training with behavior-based feedback to transfer into desirable behaviors. But when someone's intentions are contrary to the purpose of an intervention process, we have problems. A more intrusive intervention is needed, such as one-to-one coaching.

"I already knew that."

OK, but self-efficacy — knowing what to do — is only one-third of the equation for individual success in patient safety. Next question: Do you believe what we're asking you to do for patient safety will work? (This is called response-efficacy.) And finally: Do you believe the effort we're asking you to put into patient safety is worth it? (Outcome-expectancy) A "yes" answer to each of these questions reflects ownership and authentic empowerment.

Coaching for patient safety focuses not only on imparting knowledge, but building these essential beliefs:

I can do it and it will work.

I'm motivated to make it work.

I can and want to do it.

I want to make a difference.

These beliefs are inherent in the natural altruism healthcare professionals possess. Coaching, particularly through one-on-one conversation, draws out these beliefs and holds them to the light of day. In Chapter 4 on Thinking, we'll discuss building a belief system that benefits patient-safety values.

"That won't work here."

Healthcare systems are complex connections of microunits. Every nursing unit or department is its own business operation, one nurse told us. Focus on the environmental, behavioral, and personal factors that contribute to errors at the unit level. Open and frank communication within a small group of people can identify problems and solutions. Keep in mind the tone of these conversations and degree of candor are set by unit leadership.

5 How to start a patient-safety epidemic
Identify your Mavens, Connectors and Salespeople

OK, now for an antidote to fear, fatalism, fog, frustration and myths. In the national bestseller, *The Tipping Point*,[26] author Malcolm Gladwell describes how to deliberately start and control a positive emotional epidemic — such as support and participation in patient-safety efforts.

The "safety bug" can spread through your system or microsystem like a virus. And like a virus, it's based on human contact. But success in tipping patient-safety participation in the direction you want depends on three factors: 1) Your "agents of infection"; 2) the message being carried; and 3) the work environment or culture that, in effect, incubates the virus.

Let's study each of these "tipping" factors.

Carriers

To spread an epidemic, agents of infection take the form of three personality types described by Gladwell as Connectors, Mavens, and Salespeople.

Connectors are gregarious extroverts who roam the floors and have a knack for chatting it up with secretaries, transporters, lab techs, VPs, the FedEx guy. They know everyone by name. And they wield social power.

Mavens are experts, the teachers in the workplace. They don't possess the raw transmission power of Connectors. Their influence comes from collecting and brokering information that no one else possesses. Mavens are master verbal communicators.

Salespeople possess the power of persuasion, largely through non-verbal means — call it charisma, energy, presence.

To transmit a patient-safety message, to build a Patient-Safety Culture, you need all three of these agents working on your behalf.

Patient-safety officers naturally slip into the role of Maven. Mavens are "pathologically helpful" with no personal agendas, according to Gladwell. Of course that often limits their clout in the organization.

Patient-safety officers might also be Connectors. After all, their work takes them from unit to unit, into every corner of a healthcare system. Still, to generate real transmission power, they need the help of other Connectors.

You don't usually find Salespeople toiling away in patient-safety departments. What motivates most Salespeople — money and status, for instance — are not the customary currency of patient-safety work. But you need to connect to Salespeople to get your message sold. They often can be found behind clean desktops in carpeted suites.

Target your interventions

Connectors, Mavens and Salespeople are your carriers. Agents of infection. Models who give both "thumbs up" for patient safety. The few who have the power to give permission to the many. Patient safety is OK, it's the thing to do. Target your interventions, your resources, at these three groups.

Don't try to win over every single employee in your system, even in your unit, at once. Start small. Identify and cultivate your Mavens, Connectors, and Salespeople. Then turn them loose in the workplace.

This is organic growth — as opposed to required accreditation commands and organizational control through compliance.

Making it stick

What is the message you want Connectors, Mavens and Salespeople to buy into and spread? Most important, how are you going to make that message stick?

Stickiness is a problem in safety in general, due to a barrage of competing corporate messages. This is particularly true for patient safety, still in a fragile state of early development in many healthcare cultures. Posters, pep talks, banners, slogans and PowerPoint presentations don't stick — they don't leave lasting impressions. Patient-safety messages can't be allowed to drift off like the haze of a Super Bowl halftime show.

Pay attention to packaging and delivery. After all, accreditation-based patient-safety goals and requirements, well intentioned as they are, are hardly irresistible. To the contrary, they can breed indifference. Still, we've learned from general industry that many safety and health pros are blinded by the "rightness" of their message and neglect the power of packaging and embedding it.

In following chapters we discuss in detail many of the ideas promoted in *The Tipping Point* to make your message stick:

• Tell stories. Stories about close calls or an injured patient's insights are far more compelling than regulatory interpretations and error statistics.

• Be practical and personal. Teach staff how to incorporate patient safety into the jobs they do.

• Better yet, let them figure it out. No one knows the job better than those who do it.

• If they need help, use other staff as teachers, mentors, coaches.

• Don't overwhelm employees with too many learning objectives. Keep it simple.

• Test your messages. Hold focus groups. Do they "get it"? Are they "buying"? Why or why not?

And don't insult your audience. Smokers are not smokers out of ignorance, Gladwell writes in *The Tipping Point*.[27] They know the risks; they've been warned for years. The same is true in healthcare. The potential for error and harm was recognized long ago. "None of us come to work intending to kill someone," says one nurse.

Covering the basics of risk recognition is a given (see Chapter 5). Beyond that, focus on the social rules and rituals of your culture that make taking risks acceptable. As we detailed in barriers to improved patient safety, some of the most common reasons for ignoring "the right thing to do" have nothing to do with awareness, but rather fear, fatigue, frustration and fatalism.

Case Study *Organic team development at The Johns Hopkins Hospital*

Lori A. Paine, R.N., M.S., is Patient-Safety Coordinator for The Johns Hopkins Hospital.

We encourage development of Comprehensive Unit-Based Safety Program teams. First they have to define who the team is. That's easy in an ICU or OR. The boundaries are fairly clear and you have dedicated staff such as an intensivist, pharmacist, or respiratory therapist.

Applied to floor units, team membership is not black and white. In intermediate care between the floor and the ICU, how do we define physician membership? We have eight services on this unit, such as pulmonary or gastroenterology.

My advice is to find a leader, say a chief resident, who is very enthused about the potential for teams. Build your team around these leaders and the team will grow organically. And teams need to be multi-disciplinary. Our system is built on interdependency, and teams help pharmacists and nurses and physicians interact and communicate with each other.

We strive for organic growth of teams. We'd like development to come not through mandates but by having success build upon success, with teams making rounds, assessing risks, finding and fixing defects. You obtain more acceptance this way.

You can run into resistance when one unit challenges the success of another's team, saying, "That's fine but it won't work here." Anyone who's worked in clinical care knows about silos. How Unit A can be uniquely different than Unit B. One ICU is a big, happy family and a second one is filled with conflict and tension. It is important to understand and respect the unique culture of each unit.

There's nothing more frustrating than working with a team that doesn't believe in what they're doing. I'll deliver the first "science of safety" talk and their faces go blank. I'll hear, "JCAHO said I had to be here." Or "What's so new about this? We've known these things since we first put on uniforms."

That's when I show a slide titled, "How did we get here?" Our current systems have morphed from old, broken systems, with Band-Aids on top of Band-Aids. You end up with a tangled web of patient-safety problems that can be quite overwhelming. After 125 years of cumulative denial you can't see the forest, the system problems, for the trees, the immediate crises.

You have to start somewhere — with units, individual champions, and small wins. We can't use a lack of benchmarks, a lack of metrics or validated outcome data, as excuses for doing nothing.

6 How to activate ACTS

Acting, Coaching, Thinking and Seeing — The heart of People-Based Patient Safety™

At the heart of People-Based Patient Safety™ lies ACTS: Acting, Coaching, Thinking and Seeing. In a Patient-Safety Culture, people Act to prevent risk and patient harm, Coach one another to identify barriers to safe acts and provide constructive behavior-based feedback, Think in ways that activate and support safe behavior, and remove perceptual blinders to See hazards. These four essentials of People-Based Patient Safety™ — ACTS — provide knowledge, skills, and tools to fully address the human side of patient safety.

In ACTING (Chapter 2), we take a closer look at behavior — actions — and simple strategies to make sure our actions are safe.

People-Based Patient Safety™ focuses on what people do, analyzes why, and then applies a research-supported intervention strategy. The improvement results from acting people into thinking differently, rather than targeting internal awareness or attitudes so as to think people into acting differently.

Start with a behavioral analysis of work practices to pinpoint many external factors that encourage at-risk behavior.

Next, direct with activators and motivate with consequences. Activators (or signals preceding behavior) are only as powerful as the consequences supporting the behavior. Activators tell us what to do in order to receive a pleasant consequence or avoid an unpleasant consequence. Remember "A" for activator, "B" for behavior, and "C" for consequence. This principle is used to design interventions for improving behavior at individual, group, and organizational levels.

People's actions can be objectively observed and measured before and after an intervention process is implemented. This application of the scientific method provides critical feedback to build improvement.

The acronym "DO IT" says it all:

D – Define the target action to increase or decrease;

O = Observe the target action during a pre-intervention baseline period to identify natural environmental and interpersonal factors influencing it, and to set improvement goals;

I = Intervene to change the target action in desired directions; and

T = Test the impact of the intervention procedure by continuing to observe and record the target action during and after the intervention program.

In COACHING (Chapter 3), we show you techniques central to error prevention: monitoring and teamwork.

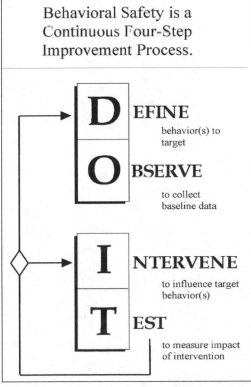

Behavioral Safety is a Continuous Four-Step Improvement Process.

DEFINE
behavior(s) to target

OBSERVE
to collect baseline data

INTERVENE
to influence target behavior(s)

TEST
to measure impact of intervention

Everyone coaches for patient safety — managers and frontline workers alike. Everyone learns the principles and procedures of behavior-based observation and feedback.

Why? Because coaching develops the self-directed accountability needed for long-term impact. Coaches feel obligated to adopt the principles and procedures they teach and advocate. To be sure, it might be necessary to start a coaching process with a select number of staff. It depends on your culture, especially the level of interpersonal trust that exists. But it's expected that eventually all employees will coach each other for injury prevention.

People-Based Patient Safety™ teaches and advocates both "formal" and "informal" coaching. Formal coaching parallels the standard behavior-based safety application of a critical behavior checklist and the DO IT process. Informal coaching involves brief personal conversations to maintain daily attention to safe and risky behaviors and conditions throughout a workplace.

By focusing more on the process of coaching than outcome checklists and numbers, you increase the quantity and quality of informal coaching. This leads to self-coaching, which is essential to the development of safe acting, thinking, and seeing of caregivers working alone.

In THINKING (Chapter 4), we show how to increase mindfulness and self-accountability for patient safety through beliefs, feedback and self-talk.

The rationale we provide ourselves for performing safe behavior determines whether we feel self-accountable and will continue to perform that behavior in the absence of an external accountability system. And of course the rationale for our behavior is determined by our thinking or self-talk. People-Based Patient Safety™ teaches the kind of thinking needed to develop self-accountability, as well as the kinds of environmental/management conditions/systems needed to promote and support self-accountability thinking.

In SEEING (Chapter 5), we walk through the basics of how to become more observant and see hazards that put patients at risk.

We cannot assume other people see what we see and interpret hazards and risk-taking as we do. People-Based Patient Safety™ teaches empathy — the need to assess the perceptions of individuals in a work group or culture targeted for an injury-prevention intervention. These perceptions are carefully considered when customizing an intervention process.

People-Based Patient Safety™ also teaches techniques for risk assessment. These include: a) appropriate alternating between focusing and scanning; b) the Exposure-Severity-Probability (ESP) approach to risk assessment; and c) the development and application of a Critical Behavior Checklist.

FAQ *What should be the goal for patient-safety initiatives? Zero adverse events?** *

It is critical to distinguish between purpose (or vision) and goals. The vision is zero adverse events, errors, or injuries to patients. This vision remains at zero regardless of daily events. Even if an error occurs or a patient is injured, the vision or purpose for healthcare activity is zero.

In contrast, the things done to prevent errors and injuries to patients reflect process. These are achievements needed on a daily basis to reach zero. We set process goals to activate and motivate these daily activities.

Use the acronym SMART to define process goals. In other words, appropriate process goals should be Specific (S), Motivational (M), Achievable (A), Relevant (R), and Trackable (T). An achievable goal is challenging but doable ("I can do it"), a relevant goal is one that connects directly to the vision of zero errors or injuries ("It will work"), and a motivational goal is one that reflects desirable and cost-effective consequences or outcome expectancies ("It is worth it"). Getting employees to state affirmatively "I can do it," "It will work," and "It's worth the effort" is the key to unlocking true empowerment.

SMART goals activate performance relevant to achieving the vision. They also motivate action because they imply consequences. These goals should be made public, and progress toward meeting certain goals should also be publicly displayed. And when progress goals are reached, a consequence should occur that recognizes the goal attainment. This could simply be a public announcement or letter from a respected individual, or it could be a group celebration.

---

*Throughout *The Anatomy of Medical Error*, at the close of each chapter, these *Frequently Asked Questions* represent an exchange between authors Scott Geller and Dave Johnson, with Dave posing the question and Dr. Geller providing the response.

CHAPTER 2 *Acting*

In this chapter you'll learn:

1 Why patient-safety improvement starts by studying behavior

Actions are critical to reducing errors and improving care

The Acting part of People-Based Patient Safety™ focuses on behavior. When addressing the human dimension of safety, why start with behavior? Because actions, as you'll see in the following examples, are simply critical to reducing errors and improving care.

"Getting it" behaviors

How do we describe someone who "gets it" when it comes to patient safety? What are the clues, where's the evidence?

Actions speak to us most clearly. Interviews for this book uncovered "getting it" behaviors such as:

Disclosure. A biomed technician knocks on the door of his department head and proceeds to inform him about a mistake he made that resulted in near harm to a patient. "He just wanted me to know. He felt he was just doing his job," recalls the manager.

Reporting. A young, nervous staffer takes his concerns about patient safety to the top, to the president of a major metropolitan hospital. "I had vetted my concerns with people I trusted. I knew I had the backup of key people," he recalls. He also had models of behavior to follow, two physicians in particular who had challenged authority in the organization without punitive consequences.

Sharing stories and a willingness to look vulnerable, perhaps even weak. In the midst of a Morbidity and Mortality conference, a first-year resident stands up and volunteers, "This is my case" while a colleague dissects a significant adverse event.

Reaching out. A clinical care specialist in the Northwest who coaches and counsels patients with chronic illnesses talks to one patient with Type 2 diabetes every day because his blood-sugar count is way high. After seven weeks, her persistence pays off. The man's blood-sugar drops from an A1c of 11 percent to 7 percent. (By the way, according to a survey conducted by the American Association of Diabetes Educators, only 24 percent of people with diabetes knew their A1c levels.)[1]

"Stopping the line," to use a quality management phrase from industry. A hospital in the Midwest averages about a dozen such stoppages a year. "Can I see you outside?" a nurse asks a physician in one case. "That's not the same color medicine you gave my son yesterday," says a mother in another. When a procedure comes to a halt, staff must verify that what was about to occur was correct.

Crossing lines of authority to speak up. A transporter mentions to a unit's head nurse, "The blood I delivered yesterday had different tags on it for this patient. What do you think?" A security guard observes a shadowy figure circling about in the hospital's parking garage one evening. He could be searching for his car, waiting for family, or who knows, carrying a weapon. The guard decides to find out. A mother of a patient notices the wrong wristband was put on her son's hand.

Modeling. A hospital administrator attending an out-of-town conference receives a call in his hotel room one evening and learns a wrongful death, a medical mistake, occurred earlier that day. He packs quickly and takes a flight home that night, and calls a meeting in his office at seven the next morning. "We didn't accomplish a lot in that meeting, but it sent a message about the seriousness of patient safety," he explains.

JCAHO behavior-oriented goals

Taking action is also inherent in the national patient-safety goals set in recent years by the Joint Commission on Accreditation of Healthcare Organizations (JCAHO), including these:

"Read back" — To improve communication among caregivers, a staff person receiving verbal or telephone orders or critical test results phoned in, verifies the complete order or test result by reading it back. (Goal 2A – JCAHO 2006 Critical Access Hospital and Hospital National Patient Safety Goals)

"Hand-offs" — To tighten up the quality and effectiveness of information and patient transfers, staff implements a standardized approach, including the opportunity to ask and respond to questions. (Goal 2E – JCAHO 2006 Critical Access Hospital and Hospital National Patient Safety Goals)

"Hand hygiene" — Staff are to comply with current Centers for Disease Control and Prevention (CDC) hand-hygiene guidelines to reduce the risk of healthcare-associated infections. (Goal 7A – JCAHO 2005 Hospital National Patient Safety Goals)

"Time out" — Before starting any surgical or invasive procedure, staff conducts a final verification process, such as a "time-out," to confirm the correct patient, procedure and site, using active — not passive — communication techniques. (Goal 1A – JCAHO 2004 Hospital National Patient Safety Goals)

"Fall prevention" — Hospitals are to implement a program to reduce the risk of patient harm resulting from falls. (Goal 9B – JCAHO 2006 National Patient Safety Goals)

"Patient engagement" — Staff in labs, home care services, disease-specific care, and assisted living care are to define and communicate the means for patients to report concerns about safety, and encourage them to do so. (Goal 13A – JCAHO 2006 National Patient Safety Goals)

Behavior-related best practices

Patient-safety best practices are often action-oriented. For example:

• "Keep workspaces where medications are prepared clean, orderly, well-lit, and free of clutter, distraction, and noise." — National Quality Forum Safe

Practice #27 (from the list of 30 safe practices endorsed by the NQF)

• "Deploy Rapid Response Teams" — one of six interventions recommended by the Institute for Healthcare Improvement in its 100,000 Lives Campaign, which aims to prevent 100,000 avoidable patient deaths by June 2006.

• "Never Leave Your Wingman" — A program of Sentara Healthcare in Norfolk, Virginia, borrows behavioral practices that have proved effective in aviation safety to teach employees to be fully engaged with one another. "Never Leave Your Wingman" stresses double-checking routine decisions and processes, talking and sharing information. A staff person never just signs off on something and leaves without asking if there are any questions and double-checking that all instructions are understood.

Classic nursing behaviors

The idea we would need patient-centered care or error reduction or safety cultures, even a system called healthcare, didn't exist in Florence Nightingale's day. But her seminal observations of nursing, "Notes on Nursing — what it is and what it is not," published in 1859, stress the need for a broad range of careful, conscientious behaviors. Be observant, quiet, punctual, polite, a clear reporter, light and steady on your feet. Maintain eye contact with patients. Preserve cleanliness.[2]

Or in her own words: Avoid "the timid, uncertain touch," she wrote.[3] "Always sit down when a sick person is talking business to you, show no signs of hurry, give complete attention and full consideration…"[4] "Every nurse ought to be careful to wash her hands very frequently during the day."[5] "…it must never be lost sight of what observation is for. It is not for the sake of piling up miscellaneous information or curious facts, but for the sake of saving life and increasing health and comfort."[6]

Almost 150 years later, Florence Nightingale's book reads like a primer on patient-centered care.

2 This is not "behavior modification"
That's a top-down, controlling and manipulative term

We believe strongly that when it comes to the human side of patient safety, whether you use training, feedback, adverse event analysis, coaching, or incentives to make improvements and reduce medical errors, first and foremost you should focus on what your people are doing. Whatever the intervention approach, above all else focus on behavior. Why?

Actions we've just described project themselves with clarity, in black and white, so to speak. You are either doing these things, or you're not. This enables objective, fair and impersonal assessments, unlike discussions revolving around attitudes and perceptions. Safety in any work environment sooner or later will surface as an emotionally charged, sensitive issue. Drain the emotion out of it as much as you can. Separate the act from the actor, and focus on the facts. What has happened? What needs to happen? What needs to be corrected?

And let's make one thing clear from the start, we're not talking about behavior modification. That's a top-down, controlling and manipulative term we find insulting. It does not reflect the behavioral principles of People-Based Patient Safety™.

But the fact is "behavior modification" is used all too often as a buzz word for safety improvement. Some people use the term to refer to the observation-and-feedback process that has been practiced in industrial workplaces since the 1970s. Others use the label to dismiss the behavior-based approach in favor of strategies that sound better, like improving attitudes, building awareness, changing culture, and optimizing systems.

The broad principles of People-Based Patient Safety™ do address management systems, as well as the inner dimensions of people such as attitudes and beliefs. (See Chapter 4 – Thinking.) Using people-based principles appropriately builds feelings of self-effectiveness, personal control, optimism, and interdependent teamwork.

This is key to engaging staff in patient safety, where the first questions often are: "What can I do?" and "Is it worth it?" We'll discuss interventions to boost attitudes and beliefs about patient safety in the chapters on Coaching, Thinking and Seeing — the other components of

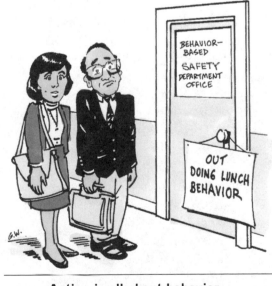

Acting is all about behavior.

ACTS, the name we give for the process of implementing People-Based Patient Safety™.

3 The Activator-Behavior-Consequence principle

Dissecting why we do what we do

The process to protect patients from harm must start with understanding why people do what they do. You simply will not be able to embed the kinds of proactive safety actions called for in patient-safety best practices, and by Florence Nightingale more than 145 years ago, unless you grasp why we do the things we do. Why sometimes we take risk and shortcuts. Why other times we are cautious and deliberate.

The basic model for understanding behavior involves: Activator-Behavior-Consequence.

The Activator comes before we act. We can design activators specifically to encourage certain behaviors or discourage others. You have to think no further than red-and-white "STOP" signs or the intent of red, yellow and green crossing lights at intersections.

A number of hospitals we contacted now use patient-safety icons that pop up on computer screens or bulletin boards. Their function: to direct staff attention to safety reminders, policies and directives. Hand-washing signs in scrubbing areas are visual cues calling for action. JCAHO's national safety patient goals are activators.

Data can serve as critical activators for patient-safety interventions. Says one nurse: "A key step to preventing failure-to-rescue events is the ability of the hospital to identify and track its complication rates. Collect and evaluate discharge data and then formulate performance improvement plans based on that data. This could provide better patient outcomes.

"It's far better to prevent a complication than it is to rescue a patient from a complication."

But activators can also be unintentional and unplanned:

• Staff members are seen using cell phones in restricted areas, sending the wrong signal.

• A patient crashes, his cardiologist's beeper goes off, and the physician rushes out from his son's basketball game.

• A gunshot victim is wheeled into the ER amid shouts and commotion, and priorities change immediately.

• An executive receives a distressing phone call in his hotel room about a grievous medical error and takes the next flight home.

The unpredictable and, at times, conflicting nature of activators in healthcare, which often come fast and furious, is a major challenge to the notion of standardizing certain procedures for patient safety.

After the Activator comes the Behavior, our response to the stimulus event. Keep in mind we are not automatons. We choose our response, our behavior. We can ignore cute little patient-safety icons on a computer screen just like we

Activator	→	Behavior	→	Consequence
Discussion/ Consensus		Drive the Speed Limit		Thank-You
Lecture/Film		Buckle Up		Self Approval
Policy		Lock Out Power		Peer Approval
Demonstration				Smile
Directing Feedback		Put On PPE		Motivating Feedback
Goal Setting		Use Equipment Guards		Prize or Reward
Pledge Signing		Give a Safety Talk		Reprimand
Incentive				Penalty
Disincentive		Clean Up a Spill		
Safety Sign		Remind Others to Work Safely		

Intervention strategies are classified by the ABC model.

ignore pop-up ads. We don't have to use our cell phone in an off-limits area just because we saw someone else do it. The cardiologist could have waited until the end of the quarter to leave his son's game. Data can be collected, only to collect dust. Goals can be discussed and debated in safety committee meetings, without agreement on an action plan.

Words of caution

A few words about using this model:

1) When studying what activates behavior in your environment, be careful of the claim that certain environmental cues "trigger" safe behavior. This implies that stimuli cause safety-related behavior to occur. Not true.

Some "triggers" do cause involuntary behavior. The flashing blue lights of a state trooper elicit certain emotional reactions. But drivers choose to slow down and pull over. Similarly, traffic lights do not trigger or cause intersection behavior, although they may cause an emotional rush following a driver's decision to speed through an intersection as the light changes from yellow to red.

Bottom line: There is a space between the stimulus (or activator) and voluntary behavior. Activators provide direction, but it's up to you whether to follow the direction. Your choice is largely determined by the way you perceive consequences. How important are the consequences to you? What positive consequence do you expect to gain, and/or what negative consequence do you expect to escape or avoid?

For example, what consequences does the ER staff perceive if the gunshot victim is not tended to immediately? What is the consequence perceived by the cardiologist if he doesn't quickly leave his son's game?

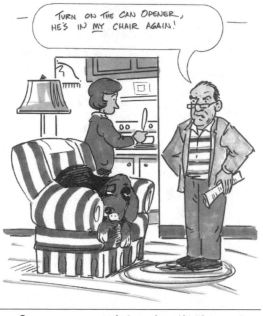

Consequences determine the impact of activators.

2) "Positive reinforcement" is an overused and abused term. A consequence reinforces positively or negatively only if it increases the behavior it follows.

Attitudes and perceptions determine the motivating potential of a reward or penalty. The reinforcing power of a consequence is in the eye of the beholder. The meaning of a safety incentive to an individual determines whether such a consequence is viewed as positive, negative, or neutral and could motivate behavior.

It's usually impossible to determine whether delivering a consequence actually influences the behavior it follows. Loose talk of "positive reinforcement" is often inappropriate. People-Based Patient Safety™ (PBPS) for patient care does not make this mistake. "Positive reinforcement" is not used in PBPS, and the impact of positive consequences on feelings, or person states, as well as behaviors is entertained and appreciated.

3) In People-Based Patient Safety™, positive consequences are considered "rewards," and negative consequences are "penalties." If these consequences don't impact overt behavior, they will at least influence feeling states, which is important in PBPS. With PBPS, rewards increase self-esteem and perceptions of personal competence and control, as well as improve behavior. Research shows these feelings increase people's willingness to actively care for the safety of others — patients, coworkers, temporary workers, visitors, etc.[7] Thus, PBPS applications of the activator-behavior-consequence model are directed to both external behaviors and internal person states.

The power of consequences

Here's an important principle to remember: the power of activators to influence behavior is determined by consequences. One of B. F. Skinner's most important legacies is "selection by consequences,"[8] which means behavior is motivated by events or conditions that follow it. Pleasant consequences can increase behavior and unpleasant consequences can decrease behavior. This is crucial for understanding why people act the way they do.

Pop psychology might say we motivate ourselves with goals or intentions, but the fact is that behavioral consequences actually motivate our activities.

Take JCAHO's National Patient Safety Goals. They carry potentially heavy consequences. Because hospitals must be accredited by JCAHO or submit to review by the Centers for Medicare and Medicaid Services in order to participate in Medicare, and with Medicare accounting for approximately 40 percent of hospitals' revenues[9], hospitals have strong motivation to meet JCAHO patient-safety requirements.

Consequences of "activating" patients

Or take efforts to "activate" patients to be more questioning and vigilant about their own health and safety. Despite the growing number of written advisories distributed to patients — brochures listing safety tips and outlining the ways patients can intervene on their own behalf — there is scant empirical evidence that these "activators" actually change patient behavior.[10] The messages are often not supported by healthcare professionals. And hospital executives often seem more interested in other types of patient-safety actions than encouraging patient involvement.

Why might activators — such as educational material — used to motivate greater patient involvement in their own care fall short of their intended impact? Why are these materials often not emphasized or supported by healthcare professionals?

Let's examine possible consequences of distributing safety tips to patients. The patient's trust in professionals might be undermined. The dissemination of these advisories might be perceived as shifting responsibility for the safety of care onto patients. On the other hand, empowering patients could lead to difficulty and more headaches for health professionals. And patients might react to advisories with guilt, labeling themselves as "bad patients" if they don't speak up or follow tips.

Taken together, these possibilities add up to a set of adverse reactions that work against activating patients. Or to put it another way, fear of negative consequences undermines efforts to empower patients.

The consequences of incident reporting

Fear of punitive or other negative consequences, and a lack of positive consequences, clearly factor into significant under-reporting of medical errors through the use of incident reporting systems.[11]

In one study of 54 medication errors detected through other means, an incident report had been completed on only three events.[12] Another study collected data on 457 medication errors; an incident report had been filed on only one.[13]

And in a survey of physicians and nurses at a children's hospital, 45.9 percent of physicians had completed zero incident reports in the previous 12 months.[14] According to the survey, only 31.3 percent of doctors and 56.9 percent of nurses completed incident reports on 80 percent or more of the errors that they themselves had committed.[15]

And respondents were even less likely to report errors committed by others. Only 37.5 percent of nurses and 33.8 percent of doctors had filed incident reports on 80 percent or more of errors that they perceived were committed by colleagues.[16]

Equally if not more discouraging, only 31.7 percent of nurses and physicians were likely or very likely to report a close call event in which a supply of breast milk is inadvertently connected to a central venous catheter — a potentially fatal medical error if completed.[18] We know from general industry experience that reporting and learning from close calls is a key element in improving safety, yet in two other hypothetical close call scenarios cited in this study less than 50 percent of nurses and physicians said they were likely or very likely to report these events.[17]

Research on incident reporting, the most commonly used method for detecting adverse patient events[19], offers us fascinating insight into how activators and consequences shape caregiver behavior relating to patient-safety improvement efforts.

In the study at the children's hospital, respondents were asked about reasons for not reporting medical errors. The number one reason: uncertainty about what is considered a medical error.[20] In other words, unclear instruction — or the lack of a precise activator for reporting. The second most-cited reason: concern about implicating others (a distinct negative consequence).[21]

"Fear prevents stepping up to report," says Martin J. Hatlie, Esq., president of the Partnership for Patient Safety in Chicago.

"You have to feel safe to report," says Lori Paine, RN, the patient-safety coordinator for The Johns Hopkins Hospital. "There can be no harassing in the parking garage."

What types of activators or consequences might increase reporting of medical errors?

• Better education about what is considered a medical error that should be reported (cited by 65.4 percent of respondents in the children's hospital survey).

• Regular feedback regarding types of frequencies of reported errors (63.8 percent).

• Evidence that reporting of errors led to systems changes (55.4 percent).

These activators and consequences were seen as having relatively little effect on increasing reporting:

• Reward for reporting medical errors (cited as likely to increase reporting by only 8.7 percent of respondents).

• Make reporting of errors mandatory (21.3 percent).

• Confidentiality — reports not directly relayed to supervisors (20.0 percent).

• Anonymity (30.7 percent).[22]

(We will have more to say about the critical importance of providing regular feedback in Chapter 3 on Coaching.)

Use of incentives: We agree with the survey respondents — an extra financial incentive should not be linked to completing medical error reports. But a recognition process for useful reports would be motivational and could activate more quality reports of close calls. Employees should complete reports on company time and receive their standard compensation. Or, if completing a report requires overtime, they should be justly compensated as for any task that takes overtime to accomplish.

Close calls: It's critical for healthcare workers to see visible consequences of completing close-call reports. A healthcare worker could get a feedback letter or interpersonal recognition that acknowledges extra effort in completing a report. Group meetings could discuss the value of close-call reporting and point out beneficial consequences. But of course, the most powerful consequence indeed would be evidence — a visible change in the environment or healthcare protocol that resulted from a close-call report.

Mandatory reporting: We agree — reporting should not be mandatory or a condition of employment. This could not only put people in the mindset of "failure avoiding," but will likely also result in incomplete reports. The ideal report includes environmental, behavioral, and personal factors that potentially contributed to the close call. This includes behaviors and attitudes of the person who experienced the event. For this to happen, people must trust the process and believe it will improve patient safety. They must own up to their own errors and seek ways to reduce them.

Owning up and self-evaluation are unlikely in a culture of mandates and conditions of employment. The motivation for such reporting should be the realization the reports lead to improvement in patient care. The real reward for these reports is seeing change resulting from the reports. Again, we're back to the importance of evidence — environmental changes, behavioral changes, or even attitudinal changes reflected in interpersonal conversation or perception surveys.

Expert Q&A
Confronting the risk of reporting

Jeffrey B. Cooper, Ph.D., is a patient-safety pioneer. His 1978 paper, "Preventable Anesthesia Mishaps: A study in human factors," was the first in-depth, scientific look at errors in medicine, based on analysis of 359 errors. Today, Dr. Cooper is director of biomedical engineering for Partners HealthCare System, Inc.; associate professor of anesthesia at Harvard Medical School; and executive director of the Center for Medical

Simulation in Cambridge, Massachusetts.

Q *At one point in your career you took your concerns about patient safety straight to the top, to the president of the hospital that employed you at the time. What enabled you to take the risk to report your concerns?*

A *I was nervous and had trepidation. But I had vetted my concerns with people I trusted. I knew I had the backup of key people.*

Also, there were two iconoclastic physicians in anesthesiology who were outspoken, sometimes to the point of being rude, but they said what they thought. They were very challenging, very demanding. But they weren't fired for challenging authority. The chair of the department tolerated them. He didn't encourage them, but he didn't try to shut them up. They drove him nuts. Those two guys caused me great anxiety and grief, but they also emboldened me. They taught me that in this environment it was OK to speak up.

4 How to set SMART goals
Specific, Motivational, Achievable, Relevant and Trackable

Goal setting is important to realizing desired patient-safety-related behavior, but only if you go about it correctly. Holding people accountable for numbers (outcomes) they do not believe they can control is a sure way to produce negative stress or distress. Some people won't be distressed because they won't take these goals seriously. Experience has convinced them they cannot control the numbers, so they simply ignore the goal-setting exhortations.

What do goals such as zero nosocomial infections or zero medication errors mean, anyway? Are these goals reached when no infections or errors are recorded for a day, a month, six months, a year? Does an infection or a medication error indicate failure? And does the average frontline caregiver believe he or she can influence goal attainment?

You can remember the techniques for setting effective goals with the SMART acronym: "S" for specific, "M" for motivational, "A" for achievable, "R" for relevant, and "T" for trackable.

SMART goal setting defines what will happen when the goal is reached, and tracks progress toward achieving the goal. Feedback from completing intermediate steps toward the ultimate goal motivates continued progress. Of course, it's critical that those asked to work toward the goal "buy in" or believe in the goal, and believe they have the skills and resources to achieve it.

Patient-safety goals should focus on process activities that can contribute to prevention of harm. Staff needs to discuss what they can do to improve patient safety and reduce errors, from reporting and analyzing "near misses" to conducting safety rounds that audit environmental conditions and certain work practices. And these activities barely scratch the surface.

In industry, we're familiar with a safety steering committee that wanted to increase daily interpersonal communications regarding safety. They set a goal for their group to achieve 500 safety communications within the following month. To do this they had to develop a way to measure and track safety communications. They designed a wallet-sized "SMART Card" for recording communications with people about safety. One member of the work team volunteered to tally and graph the daily card totals.

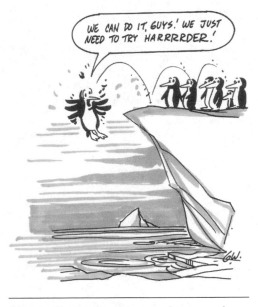

"Best efforts are not enough — you have to know what to do." W. Edwards Deming

Another work group set a goal of 300 behavioral observations of lifting. Employees had agreed to observe each other's lifting behaviors according to a critical behavioral checklist they had developed. If each worker completed an average of one lifting observation per day, the group would reach their goal within the month.

Each of these work groups reached their safety goals within the expected time period, and as a result they celebrated their "small win" at group meetings, one with pizza and another with doughnuts.

Lessons learned:

1) Apply your SMART goals to position safety as process-focused and achievement-oriented — not the standard and less effective outcome-focused and failure-oriented approach promoted with incident- or error-based goals.

2) Solicit employees to suggest relevant goals, rather than rely on more typical and less effective top-down goal setting.

3) Giving staff ownership of safety-related goals keeps them motivated to stay engaged in the safety process because it was their idea.

4) Fuel motivation to work on safety processes by keeping score of small wins — post and otherwise communicate ongoing performance results so everyone can track their ongoing achievements and estimate when they will cross the "finish line."

5 The appropriate use of discipline

Ask yourself these seven questions...

We rely too much on punishment to correct behavior. Errors, or cognitive fail-ures and mistakes (that result from our mental processes involving awareness and judgment), are unintentional and often caused by system factors. And even when errors are intentional (as in taking calculated risks), the person didn't intend to cause harm. Rather one or several environmental factors influenced the decision to take the risk. Reasons for errors and calculated risks need to be uncovered and addressed.

Before meting out punishment, answer the following seven questions. In most cases, you'll find another type of corrective action is more appropriate.

1) Was a specific rule or regulation violated?

If you answer "no," punishment is obviously unfair. Does this mean you need to write more rules or document more regulations? We don't think so. You can't write a rule for every possible at-risk behavior. And since human errors are largely unintentional, rules won't decrease them. We need to allow for the possi-bility that non-compliance with a rule or regulation can be unintended. This leads to the next question.

2) Was the behavior intentional?

Psychologists call cognitive failures or "brain cramps" slips or lapses, and they are typically due to limitations of attention, memory, or information processing.[23]

Have you ever walked into a room and forgotten why you were there? Locked yourself out of your car with the keys still inside? Left your house only to return to get something you forgot?

In work settings, research has shown these types of errors increase with expe-rience on the job. Skilled people put their actions on "automatic pilot" and perhaps add other behaviors to the situation. In healthcare, who doesn't multi-task? Every day, many of us rummage for a CD or scroll through our cell-phone directory while driving. You can see how an error can easily occur. This "unconscious incompetence" needs to be corrected, but certainly not through punishment.

There is also "conscious incompetence." Sometimes poor judgment results in intentional risk-taking. This conscious behavior can be classified as either a mistake or a calculated risk. Have you ever miscalculated a parking space and scraped an adjacent vehicle? Pressed the brake pedal too quickly on a slippery road or pumped the brakes in an antilock system? Parking and braking are frequent and intentional driving behaviors, but under particular circumstances they can be mistakes.

Now suppose you don't buckle your safety belt. You know this behavior is unsafe, but you decide to take a calculated risk. In this case, unlike a mistake, you're aware that your behavior is inappropriate. The deliberate or willful aspect of calculated risks might seem to warrant punishment, but punishment won't convince people their judgment was defective. And that's what is needed to change conscious incompetence to conscious competence.

3) Was a rule knowingly violated?

Researchers have proposed the more knowledge or skill we have at doing something, the less likely we are to demonstrate poor judgment.[24] So the driving mistakes listed above occur more often from inexperience or poor training. On the other hand, the tendency to take a calculated risk increases with experience on the job. This is human nature, and it won't be changed with punishment.

Some errors occur because the rule or proper safe behavior was not known. And it's possible for an experienced professional to forget or inadvertently overlook a rule. Training and behavior-based observation and feedback can reduce these types of errors, but punishment certainly won't help.

4) Was the harm intentional?

In industry, we've heard many safety professionals say they only punish employees when a particular behavior risks a severe injury or fatality, or places many individuals in danger. Some pros are quick to add that these risks must involve willful intentions and prior knowledge.

In healthcare, if an employee willingly and knowingly avoids a recognized patient-safety procedure that puts the patient at risk of harm, then the severest punishment is relevant Actually, this person should be discharged, have licenses revoked or restricted, or other discipline imposed immediately. But this rationale for risky behavior is very rare.

Many dangerous behaviors are mistakes resulting from poor judgment, not an unconscious or conscious desire to circumvent policies and hurt someone. And when a calculated risk is taken, it's not with the idea someone will get hurt. Often, specific characteristics of the work system or culture enable or even encourage a calculated risk.

5) What supports the behavior?

This is the most important question of all. People don't make errors or take calculated risks in a vacuum. Poor judgment occurs for a reason. And it's important to learn why a person takes a risk. This leads to truly useful corrective action.

Did the employee lack knowledge or skills? Was peer pressure or a demanding superior involved? Did equipment design invite error with poorly labeled controls? Was the "safe way" inconvenient, uncomfortable, or cumbersome?

Let's step back and look at the culture: Is safety taken seriously only after a patient is needlessly harmed? Is patient-safety performance judged only in terms of incidents reported per month, instead of the number of preventive activities?

These are only some of the questions that need to be asked. Punishment will only make resolution — a complete analysis of the situation and a practical corrective action plan — more difficult.

6) How frequent is the behavior?

How many at-risk behaviors typically occur before leading to an incident in which a patient is harmed? In industry, H. W. Heinrich estimated 300 near-misses per one major injury,[25] and Frank Bird observed this ratio to be 600 to one.[26] Both Heinrich and Bird presumed numerous at-risk behaviors occur before even a near-hit is experienced, let alone harm.

So, what good is it to punish one of hundreds of risky behaviors? If the behavior is an unintended error (not willful or knowing), punishment will only stifle reporting and potential remedies. If the probability of getting caught while taking a calculated risk is low, any threat of being punished will have little behavioral impact. Remember, punishment reduces involvement in safety improvement efforts more than it reduces risks.

7) How often have others escaped punishment?

To punish someone for a behavior that others have performed without receiving similar punishment is one sure way to lose credibility and turn a person against your safety efforts.

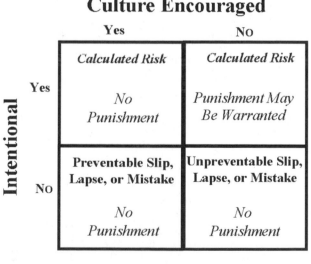

Culture Encouraged

	Yes	No
Yes (Intentional)	*Calculated Risk* *No Punishment*	*Calculated Risk* *Punishment May Be Warranted*
No (Intentional)	**Preventable Slip, Lapse, or Mistake** *No Punishment*	**Unpreventable Slip, Lapse, or Mistake** *No Punishment*

When is punishment for at-risk behavior warranted?

To summarize: If the danger of patient harm is not sufficient to motivate consistent safe behavior, it doesn't help to add one more threat (punishment) to the situation. We need open and frank discussions with people working at-risk in order to analyze and change system practices, equipment or management decisions that contribute to much of the at-risk behavior we see in healthcare settings. This is only possible when the threat of punishment is removed.

6 How to analyze safety problems by studying activators and consequences

Solve patient-safety problems by putting the pieces together

The activator-behavior-consequence principle is a good starting point for addressing patient safety issues because it pulls together for analysis loose ends of a very fragmented and compartmentalized healthcare system. It's like fitting the pieces of a puzzle together. Organize for review the intended and unintended activators, the positive and negative consequences, and the range of response patterns relevant to patient safety in your unit. Your study will help uncover why errors are occurring and patients are being harmed, or nearly so.

We hope you now see how behavior — be it error reporting, hand-offs, acting when you see something is not right, or interacting with patients — is influenced by many system-based activators and consequences. Here are a few: patient-staff ratios, work hours, goals, policies, communications, management priorities, equipment design, fear of punitive measures or loss of autonomy, and the behavior modeled by others. The list goes on and on.

One of the first steps to building a culture that truly values patient safety is to openly discuss system and interpersonal influences. Analyze in a group discussion the activators and consequences that shape patient-safety practices in your unit or department. Keep your focus narrow in the beginning, limited to one work area (or microsystem) or one problem. Piecing the puzzle together — figuring out why errors are occurring — leads to analysis that informs best practices for corrective action. Study just one significant patient-safety-related problem, for instance, and examine activators and consequences of relevant behaviors. This is a good way to keep your discussions structured and anchored.

Improving infection control

For instance, a discussion might center on this issue: Infection rates are being driven up due to a lack of compliance with accepted infection control practices. Why? And what can be done about it?

After all, a well-publicized study in the *Annals of Internal Medicine* found doctors adhered to hand-hygiene recommendations on average only 57 percent of the time. Internists were most likely to follow recommendations — they did so 87 percent of the time. Anesthesiologists adhered to guidelines only 23 percent of the time.[27]

Perhaps most disturbing was the finding that hand-hygiene adherence (use of gloves, failure to remove gloves after contact, handwashing and hand-rubbing) was lowest when doctors were performing activities considered to be at the highest risk for contaminating the patient — such as surgery or treating patients in the ER.[28]

A frontline nurse we interviewed provided answers to the low compliance rates, putting it in terms of consequences. "The percentages are low for the same reason most people don't wash their hands: it's just too much trouble. Hand-washing is time-consuming and inconvenient. Sinks are often placed far from where actual care is being rendered."[29]

She is on the money, of course. According to the Annals of Internal Medicine study, two out of three physicians perceived hand hygiene as a difficult task, especially physicians with a high workload.[30]

Our nurse agreed. "High workloads present challenges for staff to comply with infection control policies. Shortcuts to both hand-hygiene practices and donning personal protective equipment (PPE) often occur when the patient census is high and staff is low."

She then noted another motivating consequence: "It may not be right, but it's a reality that when a patient has a known infectious disease like HIV or Hepatitis B, the staff are more compliant with infection control practices."

In other words, when a consequence is "known" — more obvious — and especially more personally threatening, compliance increases.

When consequences are not understood, a different set of behaviors can result. Said our nurse: "Infection rates are often not communicated to the front-line worker, so they may not know or believe there is a problem with nosocomial infections in their work setting. It may be a case of 'no news is good news.' It's difficult to get staff to 'buy in' to the importance of infection control when they don't witness the effects of not doing so."

Again, she is correct. The hand-hygiene study reported doctors didn't think it was important to wash or rub after removing gloves because they did not believe their hands were dirty. [31] But it's important to clean hands after using gloves because the bacteria normally on hands will grow — it's like putting the bacteria in a warm moist environment. These bacteria will be deposited on everything touched after removing gloves.

Our nurse pointed to another consequence that limits the frequency of hand-washing — discomfort. "Frequent washing dries and chafes the skin," she explained. To counter the effects of this consequence, "alcohol-based hand rubs should be readily accessible and should be the standard of care for hand hygiene in health care settings," she said.

This brief examination of hand-hygiene tendencies in healthcare shows the value of attending to consequences (and activators) whenever you address a patient-safety issue. You'll find at-risk and unhealthy behaviors are often followed naturally by immediate and pleasant consequences — comfort, convenience, excitement, sensory stimulation. No trekking off to some remote wash station. No chafed skin.

In contrast, safe and healthy behaviors are usually accompanied by inconvenience (the time it takes to walk to that wash station), discomfort (the dry skin), or boredom ("Do I have to wash my hands again!").

Plus, the presumed benefits of safe and healthy behaviors are either not experienced — no incident or error or infection occurs to demonstrate the value of proper hand hygiene — or benefits are too delayed or uncertain to have much impact on current behavior. This is why some hospitals attempt to motivate healthy infection control practices by posting infection rates in units for all to see.

"Measurement, and holding people accountable to the numbers, are key," says Peter Perreiah, MBA, managing director of the Pittsburgh Regional Healthcare Initiative. Perreiah served as a PRHI coach at the Veteran Affairs' University Drive acute-care hospital where in post-surgical unit, 4 West, Methicillin-Resistant Staphylococcus Aureus (MRSA) infections were virtually eliminated.

"No one tracked MRSA infections here, and caregivers were shocked to learn how patients were colonized. When we were able to show infection rates going down, they could see the connection between their positive behaviors and the positive outcomes," he explains.

After educating staff on infection control protocols, Perreiah and the PRHI staff conducted observations of 1,000 patient encounters at the VA to verify change in behavior relating to infection control.

Observation data indicated — surprise! — the need to focus on gloving and hand hygiene. Perreiah and his team would then sit down with supervisors and unit members and use the data to explain current practices and show what needed to change.

Beliefs and perceptions toward hand hygiene: Let's use the *Annals of Internal Medicine* hand-hygiene survey for broader insight into the challenges of increasing compliant patient-safety behavior. For example, most of the physicians reported they were aware of the risk resulting from non-compliance (85 percent), they intended to comply (77 percent), and they were motivated to improve their compliance level (74 percent). And most (92 percent) had a positive attitude toward compliance after patient contact.[32]

So, if you have individuals who are aware, well intentioned, motivated and possessing a positive attitude regarding a desired behavior, what prevents them from following through and acting accordingly?

Here's one factor cited in the study: Only 44 percent of physicians considered they could be perceived as role models by their colleagues. "Reinforcement of the idea that each individual can influence the behavior of colleagues may prove to be a fruitful intervention," concluded the researchers.[33]

7 How to conduct observations and feedback sessions

The key: talk about what you see and learn

"If you cannot get in the habit of observation one way or other, you had better give up being a nurse, for it is not your calling," wrote Florence Nightingale in "Notes on Nursing." Without "the habit of ready and correct observation… we shall be useless with all our devotion."[34]

Working with hundreds of clients in industry, Dr. Geller has used for decades an observation and feedback process he defines by the acronym "DO IT."[35] As introduced in Chapter 1, the process involves the following four steps:

• D – Define the target behavior you want to increase or decrease;

• O – Observe the target behavior during a pre-intervention baseline period and then study trends, set behavior-change goals, and entertain natural environmental or social factors influencing the target behavior;

• I – Intervene to change the target behavior in desired conditions;

• T – Test the impact of the intervention procedure by continuing to observe and record the target behavior during the intervention program. Evaluate the cost-effectiveness of the intervention, decide whether to continue the program, implement another strategy, or define another behavior for the DO IT process.

The process begins by defining behaviors (such as removing unnecessary catheters, wearing sterile gowns, cleaning hands often and prescribing appropriate antibiotics for improved infection control). If two observers record the same frequency of a targeted behavior during the same time period, the definition is sufficient for an effective DO IT process.

The intervention phase of DO IT involves applying one or more behavior-change techniques, according to the activator-behavior-consequence principle.

Activator strategies range from communication or education procedures (lectures, policies, demonstrations, group discussions, consensus building) to others typically associated with organizational behavior management (goal setting, commitment, competition, incentives, and disincentives).

Consequence techniques follow the target behavior immediately, and thereby influence whether it occurs again. Examples: feedback, rewards, or penalties given after individual or group behavior.

Observation and intervention works. In the Annals of Medicine study, adherence to hand-hygiene guidelines was higher (61 percent) when physicians were aware of being observed than when they were not aware of being observed (44 percent).[36] They did better when they knew they could be held accountable.

Overcoming observation barriers

Infection control is one area in healthcare where behavioral observations have demonstrated a degree of effectiveness in bringing about safe behavior and reducing at-risk behavior. But hospital-acquired infections are only one of dozens of patient-safety and quality issues, and the broader application of behavioral observations in healthcare may be more restricted than in general industry.

For one thing, you need defined behaviors that occur at specific times and places for observation sessions — not always feasible given the fluid movements of caregivers. Plus, healthcare work is dynamic and subject to sudden changes in routine, compared to observing more fixed tasks in industry.

Also, many observation interventions in industry use a large pool of employees to serve as observers. Healthcare suffers from a shrinking pool of labor and employees very pressed for time.

Healthcare's hidebound hierarchies can be another barrier to observations. Do you really expect nurses to observe and critique physicians? In industry, most observations are peer-to-peer, or supervisor-to-subordinate.

Yes, these barriers are challenging. But anything preventing one-to-one conversations about behavioral improvement must be eliminated. Patient-safety improvement — any kind of improvement — absolutely requires feedback. And remember, everyone wants to do the best job at something they believe is important — whether it's patient care or anything else. This is the premise upon which a behavior-based observation program process is based.

Hierarchical barriers once existed in airplane cockpits. A copilot would not point out a potential error to a pilot, nor would a flight attendant suggest a problem to a copilot or pilot. Thankfully, this has changed. The airline industry learned the hard way. Lack of interpersonal communication about potential errors during flight operations actually contributed to plane crashes. Now, communication between all members of a flight crew, from pilot to flight attendant and from crew chief to flight officer, is more open and trusting.

Tracking behaviors

The idea of a behavioral checklist should not be unacceptable among healthcare professionals. Doctors in residence for example, follow physicians during rounds and listen to explanations for diagnosis and therapy. A behavioral checklist could be used to make these interactions more objective, comprehensive, and understandable.

Also, the progress of a patient is charted. Although data on these charts are medication- and symptom-focused, patient behaviors could also be tracked. Indeed, patient behavior may help to differentiate the diagnosis.

Using a checklist to track progress and learn ways to improve is not foreign to healthcare workers. But direct application of a checklist to assess ongoing behaviors and potential errors is rare in healthcare systems. With a little ingenuity, though, behavioral checklists could be used in a hospital setting to improve patient care.

Imagine the advantage of defining the diverse tasks of a healthcare worker on a behavioral checklist that specifies safe versus at-risk ways of completing

Expert Q&A

"It's not my job to police a physician!"

Lori A. Paine, R.N., is the patient-safety coordinator for The Johns Hopkins Hospital.

Q *What has been your experience with behavioral observations?*

A *We've had success using checklists and observations to reduce catheter-related bloodstream infection. The checklist uses CDC recommendations, very simple things like wash your hands, use specific skin preparation techniques, full body drapes. The checklist should be completed by a bedside nurse, while the physician is performing a central line insertion. If the team member prepping for the line insertion fails to complete a step and jeopardizes a sterile field, the nurse is to stop the process.*

At first, we had nursing staff say, "Whoa. It's not my job to police a physician. You're nuts. I'm not telling the doctor he is doing it wrong."

And we had physicians say, "Are you crazy? Nurses will challenge me in front of a patient?"

The answer? Frame it in moral terms. Can you watch and not act if you see something wrong? If it was your mom who was the patient, could you not act? It needs to be done by someone, by everyone.

We used the checklist as a tool to empower the nurse. They were given the phone number of the attending physician to call if there was a problem, but they never used it. As the team in ICU saw bloodstream infections nosedive, more got on board. We modified the checklist and staff wouldn't proceed without it. You couldn't start a line without someone else being there to check. In one ICU we went nearly one year without a bloodstream infection, which was previously thought to be unachievable. We watched infections drop and celebrated.

each behavioral component of a job. The training advantages of preparing such a checklist in a group setting are obvious. Healthcare workers could learn from each other the safest way of carrying out their duties, as well as become aware of potential risks. Individual input in preparing such a checklist would lead to a synergistic outcome.

But how do we implement or use the checklist after it's prepared? This is certainly a challenge in a system where people work alone or when they work with a diverse and changing team of others. Obviously, self-observation is possible for the lone worker. In other words, individuals can use a checklist to hold themselves accountable to performing their task in the safest manner. This works when people are self-accountable, but sometimes we need others to hold us accountable.

Whenever healthcare workers do a job with another person, a behavioral checklist could be used. Or whenever a physician teaches another physician, a behavioral checklist could be used. Whenever a nurse shows another nurse or nurse's aide how to care for a patient, a behavioral checklist could be used to facilitate the interpersonal training. These are only a few examples where a behavioral checklist could be used to facilitate interpersonal learning during interpersonal conversation.

The challenge is to teach everyone basic concepts of behavioral observation and feedback, and the value of improvement through interpersonal feedback. Then, people need to be involved in developing behavior-based checklists for various healthcare chores. This should be seen as a valuable learning experience.

Presenting feedback

Yes, there will be resistance to interpersonal feedback. But work with those who buy in and own the feedback process. Soon these volunteers will demonstrate the benefits of the process by their own participation, and soon others will join. It is a process of continuous improvement, and participation increases as improvement is demonstrated.

Clearly we are talking about revolutionary thought (think back to Chapter 1) and a culture change. But it should be obvious that open communication is needed for optimal healthcare. It is critical for healthcare workers to recognize the interdependency of healthcare. Everyone has a critical role to play. And each role can be improved with feedback from others. We need supportive feedback to keep doing the right thing, and we need corrective feedback to improve.

Obviously the level of feedback varies with one's expertise. A nurse cannot give feedback on certain learned skilled behaviors of physicians, and doctors cannot give feedback on certain abilities of nurses. But a behavioral checklist offers common ground for interpersonal feedback. Of course we don't

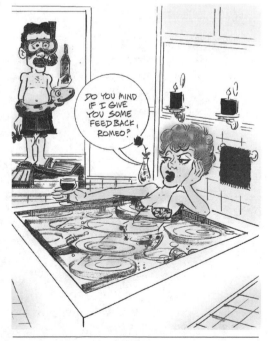

Feedback makes it possible to improve.

want to tread on the special competencies of health professionals when giving feedback. We are just considering common-ground behaviors relevant to preventing errors.

Here's another thought: It's possible to give feedback in a personal yet anonymous way on a computer database. In other words, healthcare workers could record observations on a computer spreadsheet that would be available to the hospital staff in terms of group percentages of safe behavior.

For example, Dr. Geller's students are currently evaluating potential errors in ordering and delivering medications in a hospital. Data are obtained from hospital forms and percentages of certain errors are calculated from these data. Eventually these data will be displayed to healthcare workers in an attempt to increase the use of a computer-based system, with physicians using Palm Pilots™ to order medication.

As people participate in open communication about possible errors, and see the benefits of interpersonal observation and feedback, they develop trust in the process and get more involved. Seeing is believing, and believing leads to empowerment. This takes time, but time well worth spending.

We'll cover the art of giving feedback in more depth in Chapter 3 on Coaching.

Case Study

Observation & measurement at a VA hospital

Peter Perreiah, MBA, is managing director of the Pittsburgh Regional Healthcare Initiative, a consortium of 44 hospitals, four insurers, and dozens of businesses founded in 1997 to improve healthcare for patients in southwestern Pennsylvania.

Perreiah served as a PRHI coach at the Veteran Affairs' University Drive acute-care hospital. In the hospital's post-surgical unit, 4 West, Methicillin-Resistant Staphylococcus Aureus (MRSA) infections were virtually eliminated in what PRHI calls a "confluence of patient safety and worker safety."

We needed to build confidence before pushing on safety. People were disengaged. They knew things were wrong and they couldn't get things fixed. They had lost confidence in the system healing itself.

We said we're going to improve the quality of your work life. People were always playing catch up. We said, "Tell us where your time is being wasted." We knocked out 90% of downtime in one case by fixing a computer problem. That built confidence and trust. It opened eyes. Then we moved to other complaints.

We asked, "What's a reasonable expectation for reducing MRSA?" In northern Europe, research shows it's been almost wiped out, so we could say these steps really work — patient screening, isolating patients who harbor the organism, adherence to contact precautions, having a reliable, accessible supply of hand-hygiene products, and other measures.

Staff has to perceive it's actually practical to do something like this. You need to identify cultural barriers, and you need to get a clear mandate from leaders. Also, you need clear, scripted instructions. If you see unprotected staff contacting carriers, how do you react, what do you say?

To verify change in behavior related to infection control, we conducted observations of 1,000 patient encounters at the VA. The PRHI staff did these observations. I did many myself. At Alcoa we had an observation program that was highly successful in engaging people. (Perreiah managed Alcoa's Foundry Metals business and was production system manager for Alcoa's Primary Metals business.)

Observers had a checklist of what to watch for based on CDC gloving and hand-hygiene policies and exposure and transmission pathways. We'd tell a unit that people will be observing and it's completely anonymous. We would not single out individuals but use aggregate data to identify behaviors to focus on.

Some staff were supportive and enthused about the program. They knew it's the right thing. Others were suspicious and might say something like, "I'll go back to doing what I was doing when you turn away."

Observation data told us we needed to focus on gloving and hand hygiene. We'd take these learnings, sit down with supervisors and unit members, and explain this is what we're seeing, this is what needs to change.

We admit there is a Hawthorne Effect, which makes me a little skeptical of observation data. From a baseline of 330 observations we saw pretty strong improvement in six months regarding adherence to infection control protocols. Performance was flat from six months to 18 months.

I prefer to look at glove and gown consumption versus something like a 3 percent increase in positive observations. It's common practice to use one pair of gloves for many patients, and there can be notoriously bad problems with disinfecting hands. We made supplies more accessible and saw a 30 percent increase in use of hand-hygiene products.

Still, observation data are best when they show you patterns of behavior. We've learned so much from this feedback process.

Physicians want to see journal citations before altering their behaviors, but behavior is usually not evidence-based. It's a replication of bad habits learned through mentors. So we targeted chief residents to become the teachers — got them modeling the right behavior. Some old habits die hard, so you need leaders, the chief of surgery, to say, "This will be done or come see me."

Measurement, and holding people accountable to the numbers, are key. No one tracked MRSA infections here, and caregivers were shocked to learn how patients were colonized. When we were able to show infection rates going down, they could see the connection between their positive behaviors and the positive outcomes.

The art of medicine persists only due to lack of measurement. The answer to overcoming resistance to standardized protocols is one word — measurement. Measurement is the way out. It is powerful.

8 The three basic modes of behavior
The objects of your observations

Let's consider the three types of behavior that are the focal points of observation programs, group discussions, incident analyses, and one-on-one coaching — other-directed, self-directed, and habitual actions.

Most voluntary behavior starts out as other-directed, in the sense that we follow someone else's instructions. Direction (such as an activator) can come from a training program, manual or policy statement.

A behavior-based observation-and-feedback process initiates and sustains other-directed behavior. Workers increase safe behavior and decrease at-risk behavior because others — their peers — hold them accountable.

After learning what to do, essentially by memorizing or internalizing instructions, our behavior can become self-directed. We talk to ourselves before acting, cueing memories of what we've learned to guide ourselves. At this point, we're usually open to corrective feedback if it's delivered well.

Self-directed behavior is important in healthcare, where many tasks are performed by people working alone. They need to coach themselves. This requires a sense of self-accountability. People need to believe in and own the safe way of doing things.

Self-direction requires an internal justification for the right behavior. This happens when external consequences supporting an action (such as rewards) fall short of wholly justifying the behavior. Too often people choose safe over at-risk acts only because they want to obtain a reward or avoid a penalty. These programs often get the desired behavior — while this accountability system is in place. But what happens when the external rewards or penalties are unavailable?

The key is not to over-justify safe behavior with large incentives and severe threats, but to provide education, training, and experience to help people develop a sense of personal control over preventing injuries.

Some behaviors become automatic after we perform them frequently and consistently over a period of time. Automatic behavior or a habit is formed. Some habits are good and some are not, depending on their short and long-term consequences.

Matters of habit

Of course automatic behaviors among healthcare workers vary according to job and setting. Putting a patient to sleep or making an incision is automatic for an anesthesiologist and surgeon respectively, but few of the rest of us perform these functions.

Medication administration is one automatic behavior that affects a variety of caregivers and is prone to error. The frequent task of writing or giving verbal orders, especially for familiar meds such as antibiotics, places the physician at risk of slipping up because he/she often relies on memory for a patient's history, proper doses to order, etc.

When physicians have a high patient load, it can be difficult to remember that Mrs. Jones has renal dysfunction and Mr. Smith liver dysfunction, but these distinctions are crucial due to the way drugs are metabolized by the body. Overdoses can occur even at "normal" doses if a patient can't excrete the drug properly.

Preparing and dispensing medications often becomes second nature to both pharmacists and nurses. Shortcuts might follow, such as skipping having another pharmacist or nurse check a high-risk medication (such as chemo) before dispensing or administering.

Obtaining and labeling specimens (drawing blood, for example) are frequent tasks that can cause a healthcare worker to fail to use the required two "unique identifiers" for a patient. Slip-ups occur when the specimen gets mislabeled (which obviously can be very serious for a patient). Or the specimen may fail to get labeled, delaying diagnosis and care, or at the very least, causing the patient to undergo a second stick.

Other automatic behaviors include taking vitals signs, starting and discontinuing IVs, setting alarms on equipment, transferring patients in and out of bed, prepping patients for procedures, following standard precautions such as hand hygiene and the proper use of personal protective equipment (PPE), as well as documenting care.

Bottom line: Developing safe habits is a key objective of behavioral observation processes. Daily repetition of an observation-and-feedback process builds "habit strength," eventually resulting in the development of safe habits. This is good, but not ideal.

Behavior can become so automatic in healthcare you don't notice yourself slipping across that very thin margin of error. We hope you agree self-directed or mindful behavior is more desirable than mindless, habitual behavior. We will discuss strategies to increase mindfulness more fully in Chapter 4 on Thinking.

9 Major categories of error

Know what you are looking for

Let's look at observations in another light, in terms of the errors we are attempting to catch — slips, mistakes, and calculated risks.

This is a significant challenge in patient safety: to define the types of medical errors you want to see reported by frontline caregivers. As we discussed earlier in this chapter, research at a children's hospital indicated the number one reason given by physicians and nurses for not reporting a greater number of errors was uncertainty about what is considered a medical error.[37]

The Institute of Medicine defines medical error as "the failure to complete a planned action as intended or the use of a wrong plan to achieve an aim."[38]

That leaves a lot of wiggle room for interpretation. On the other hand, one list of the types of medical mistakes itemizes 47 errors in the categories of diagnosis, treatment, prevention, surgery, hospital, medication, pharmacist, pathology lab, equipment failure, and unnecessary medical treatment.[39]

To use a behavorial term, each healthcare system should "operationalize" its definitions of medical error, replacing any vague guidelines with specific actions.

Our purpose here, though, is educational: to understand how we make errors. Let's consider how we process information. We're continually taking in a stream of information, evaluating it, and acting on our interpretations and decisions. Dr. David Bates of Brigham and Women's Hospital estimates an average internist, seeing patients from 8 a.m. to 5 p.m., makes several hundred decisions each day. Slips or lapses might occur at any point in this continuous cycle of information processing — which involves attention to a stimulus, encoding and identifying the input, using this input and memory to decide on an appropriate response, and executing the behavior.

Types of errors

Input errors. This is failure to detect, recognize, or identify. It could be because our eyesight is poor (a physical limitation) or because there is glare on a dial (an environmental condition). We can also tune out signs and warnings in a process called habituation. We're sure you've seen this in caregiving. As people become more competent and confident, they pay less deliberate attention to what they are doing. Then the potential for an input error increases.

Judgment errors. This is a matter of interpreting our sensory input and deciding on a course of action in a way that puts patients at risk.

Output errors occur while executing a task. These are risky performance-based behaviors we can readily observe. Limitations in strength, reaction time, coordination, or endurance can cause these errors, brought on by psychological or physical variables including fatigue, distress, alcohol, age, arthritis, or a cumulative trauma disorder, to name a few.

Experienced healthcare staff can err by operating on "automatic pilot." More often, though, errors of execution occur when work systems do not adequately account for human limitations and characteristics. In our stressed and strained U.S. healthcare system — with 890 million annual physician office visits,[40] 110.2 million emergency room visits annually,[41] 43.9 million inpatient procedures conducted annually,[42] and almost one-third of physicians working 60-plus hours a week [43] — it's obvious how errors of execution can occur.

Mistakes versus slips

Mistakes and calculated risks occur when a patient, a case, a situation is evaluated and a decision reached on how to act. Residents in training might make mistakes when they don't know the safe way to perform a task, or when they don't understand the need for special precautions. They might take calculated risks when they know the safest way of doing something but take a shortcut, sometimes with the perceived support from their peers. Experienced professionals make mistakes by taking safety for granted. Their skills and experiences can encourage them to take calculated risks.

Slips can be described as "brain cramps" which generally occur in the input and output stages of processing information.

Capture errors occur when actions seem dictated by familiar routines. The list of such processes in healthcare is almost endless: marking, labeling, verifying, prescribing, measuring, diagnosing, dispensing, transferring, prepping, testing, along with procedures ranging from putting patients under anesthesia and reading X-rays to taking vital signs and making incisions in surgery.

Description errors arise when the margin between correct and incorrect actions is thin. This is all too common in healthcare. Take alarm settings on monitoring equipment, for instance, or medications almost identical in name, or the placement of a decimal point in dosages. To help reduce description errors, identify processes where the margin of error is slight but unforgiving in your unit or department.

Loss-of-activation errors are commonly referred to as "forgetting." This happens whenever you start an activity — administering a med, running an IV line — with a clear goal, but then

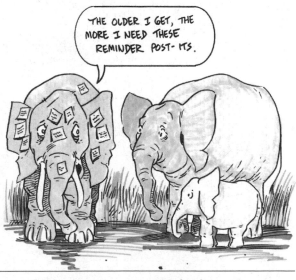

Activators can prevent brain cramps.

lose sight of it as you continue the task. You get distracted, receive a call, someone ducks in and asks a question. Performance can subsequently slip up.

We can prevent this by adding specific behavior-based activators — signs, goal-setting discussions, verbal reminders, and friendly hand gestures — to guide performance.

Mode errors are probable whenever we face a procedure involving multiple options. Not surprisingly, medical diagnoses that are wrong, missed or delayed make up a large percentage of all medical errors.[44] These errors often involve memory and interpreting information.

Talk it over

Setting up behavioral observation procedures to catch these errors is important, but the only way we can reduce their frequency is through open and frequent discussions. By revealing our own slips and mistakes in group meetings, we raise awareness of these errors and motivate others to be honest and caring.

"Just talk about it, that's the best place to start," says Julianne Morath, M.S., R.N., chief operating officer of Children's Hospitals and Clinics of Minnesota. "People in healthcare have lived so long in high-risk environments they've lost situational awareness. They've normalized the deviance."

When discussing errors, it's important to note the difference between intentional errors, as in "consciously incompetent," or unintentional errors as in "unconsciously incompetent."

This distinction is critical because it determines the nature of the intervention or corrective action to stop such errors. If the error is unintentional, education and training can work. But if the error is intentional, contingencies or consequences are needed. This could involve incentives, disincentives, or corrective coaching.

The intervention we use to improve the performance of patient care is influenced by how we define the problem. Methods to correct inappropriate behavior are different than strategies for aiding appropriate behavior. Usually the ideal approach involves both decreasing undesirable behavior and increasing desirable behavior.

Healthcare professionals work with the best of intentions. They want to do their best to reduce errors related to patient safety. They only need education, training, and behavior-based feedback to improve. But when people's intentions are contrary to the purpose of an intervention process, we have problems. A more intrusive intervention is needed, such as one-to-one coaching.

"The sin is not the mistake, but in not sharing, not disclosing what happened." — Martin Hatlie

10 How to influence behavior
Instructing, supporting and motivating

Whether you succeed in increasing safe behaviors or decreasing risky behaviors relating to a procedure, the delivery of a service, or processes in a unit, department or office, depends on many factors:
  • What behaviors are you targeting?
  • What are the personal characteristics of the individual you are coaching?
  • What is the context or environmental setting for the target behavior(s)?
  • What type of intervention strategy is called for? The impact of a particular intervention depends on the complex interplay between targeted behaviors, environmental circumstances, and personal dynamics.

Let's discuss what intervention strategies are most appropriate for influencing certain types of behavior change:

1) First we have *instructional interventions*. These typically serve to activate or direct behavior prior to it happening. (Remember, "A" represents activators or antecedent events that precede behavior, indicated by "B," and "C" is the consequence following behavior and produced by it. Activators typically direct behavior and consequences motivate behavior.)

Instructions can turn automatic habits into self-directed behaviors, or improve behavior that is already self-directed. The aim is to get an individual's attention and change unconscious incompetence into conscious competence.

Instructional intervention consists primarily of activators: education sessions, training exercises, and directive feedback. Since your purpose is to instruct, the intervention comes before the target behavior occurs, and focuses on helping the individual understand and internalize your instructions. This approach is more effective when instructions are given one-to-one. Role-playing exercises give instructors opportunities to customize directions and give feedback.

Once a person learns the right way to do something, practice is important. This is the way behavior becomes part of a natural routine. Continued practice leads to fluency and in many cases to automatic or habitual behavior.

"Practice, just doing it, builds confidence, competence, and optimism," says Julianne Morath.

2) But practice does not come easy, and can benefit greatly from *supportive intervention*. Encouragement keeps us going and reassures us we're doing the right thing.

Supportive intervention focuses on applying behavioral consequences. When we give people rewarding feedback or recognition for some particular safe behavior, we show our appreciation and increase the likelihood they will perform the behavior again.

Supportive intervention is a natural technique to use in healthcare, when professionals know what to do. This kind of support assumes the person is already motivated to do the right thing. Incentives or disincentives, promises or threats, are not needed.

3) When someone knows how to work safely but doesn't do it, *motivational intervention* is needed. In this case, the person is consciously incompetent about safety-related behavior. Instruction alone is obviously insufficient. And we don't want to support their calculated risk-taking.

Why do we take calculated risks — not double-checking, not gloving, rushing to arrive at a diagnosis? Usually it's because we perceive the positive consequences to be more powerful than the negative ones. The reasons for taking the risk — comfort, convenience, and efficiency — are immediate and certain. Doing harm, on the other hand, is improbable. In this situation, we often need to use both activators and consequences to move people from conscious incompetence to conscious competence.

An incentive/reward program attempts to motivate a certain target behavior by promising people a positive consequence if they perform it. The promise is the incentive and the consequence is the reward.

In healthcare, it's our observation that positive consequences are used much less frequently than negative consequences to motivate behavior change. Healthcare is rife with rules, policies, and the dark cloud of malpractice that threaten professionals with a negative consequence if they fail to comply, or if they take a calculated risk.

Still, this approach is often ineffective. Threats of punishment appear to challenge individual autonomy and choice. The result: less transparency in patient safety in general, less reporting of incidents, fewer opportunities to learn and eliminate the risk of future errors.

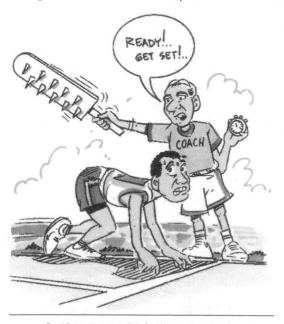

Acting to avoid failure is not fun.

Motivational intervention is clearly the most challenging of the three strategies outlined here. Remember, powerful external consequences might work — but only as long as the intervention is in place. The individual is consciously competent, but the person's behavior is not self-directed. The behavior comes from excessive outside control. It's possible a long-term motivational intervention, coupled with consistent supportive intervention, can lead to a good habit. This is how other-directed safe behavior can move to unconscious competence without first becoming self-directed.

Case study

Behavior-based expectations at Sentara Healthcare

Gary R. Yates, M.D., is the chief medical officer for Sentara Healthcare, Norfolk, Virginia.

Q *Sentara Healthcare won the 2005 Eisenberg Patient Safety and Quality Award from JCAHO and the National Quality Forum for Culture of Safety initiative. How did you drive culture change in an organization with more than 12,000 employees?*

A *In 2002 we were frustrated that as an organization we were not progressing with patient safety as quickly or as broadly as we wanted. We were beginning to have breakthroughs in ICUs with our remote patient monitoring system, for example. It was the first commercial application of the E-ICU system, developed by two doctors from Johns Hopkins. The critical care director and two nurses could monitor 95 patients across five hospitals. We saw a 20 percent relative decrease in mortality in those units.*

We had also seen improvement in medication safety with our pharmacy information system. However, what we saw in general were improvements in specific aspects of safety and quality in silos in the organization, in defined areas. But we still saw déjà vu events, the same problems over and over again. Root cause analysis would show that important communication didn't take place. A double check was not done, time and again, for example.

We decided to look at other culture-change models outside healthcare. We hooked up with Performance Improvement International, a consultancy that had improved safety at Duke Power. Their model was to work on one plant at a time. In healthcare, that would equate to one hospital. So we tried techniques first at Norfolk General. We'd watch and learn and then spread learnings throughout the organization.

Our objective was to create a culture, an environment that supported the practice of safe habits, safe behaviors. We wanted to create mindfulness. This would be an additional safety net under the system to prevent harm from reaching the patient.

As an initial assessment, we conducted a culture survey and assessed our management system. To discover weaknesses, we did a common cause analysis of 20 of our most significant events. We identified causal factors linked to these key events. Four factors were linked with 90 percent of those events — lapses in a common/repetitive task; no double-check communication; ignorance of policies and procedures, or non-compliance; and clearly obvious high-risk situations were not recognized, or the cycle of activity couldn't be halted.

We assessed behaviors linked to those four factors, and came up with a list of behaviors for employees to follow. They needed a tool to use, something more than telling them "just be more vigilant." The list of Behavior-Based Expectations (BBEs) we developed is a tool to really engage all 12,000 of our employees. They were developed by 25 employees and 14 physicians, based on dialog and data. It's critical for obtaining local buy-in, critical for employees to take ownership of these expectations, that they view them as coming from the grassroots.

Five behaviors are targeted:

• Clear communication using crew resource management concepts and phonetics when needed.

• Attention to detail by taking a moment to pause and gather your faculties, we call it STAR — Stop, Think, Act, Review.

• A readiness to question by encouraging people to speak up, to verify and validate. For example, one of our transporters mentioned the blood he delivered yesterday had a different tag on it for the same patient. "What do you think?" he asked. He caught a mistake.

• Strong, reliable hand-offs, whether they involve information or patients. All exchanges cover the 5 Ps — patient, problem, purpose, procedure and precautions.

• Something we call, "Never leave your wingman." It's a matter of being there for your coworker. Clearing you head and double-checking for them.

These five behaviors are adapted by employees to their own situations. They were customized for physicians.

We want these behaviors to become habits so they don't feel like extra work for everyone. We use plus-side motivators to encourage them. Managers go out and observe these behaviors. Safety coaches volunteer in each unit to be observers. Senior executives have BBEs built into their goals. But your real leadership is at the unit level.

We track the number of behavioral observations conducted. We share feedback monthly on what managers, observers and coaches have seen. And they will intervene immediately if they see problems.

We've seen a significant decrease in the most serious events — National Quality Forum "Never Again" events and JCAHO sentinel events, for example. These events declined 45 percent over 24 months, not just at Norfolk General but throughout our system.

We believe we're consistent in how we collect data, so the changes year-to-year are valid measures. But we're still a work in progress.

11 Correct use of incentives

Don't "over-justify" target behavior

The power of incentives or disincentives depends on the size, immediacy, and certainty of the consequences they announce. Generally, consequences are more influential motivators of behavior when they are large (a valuable reward or severe penalty), immediate (presented soon after the behavior), and certain (likely to occur after the target behavior).

Suppose external consequences are not powerful enough to fully control safe behavior all the time. Perhaps we're talking about pats on the back, coffee mugs, or other tokens. If people follow safety requirements in this situation — a big "if" sometimes — it is because they develop internal controls to justify their behavior.

Researchers have demonstrated that people are more apt to develop internal motivation when external rewards or threats are relatively small and insufficient to completely justify a target behavior. This phenomenon has been referred to as the "less-leads-to-more effect."[45] It's most likely to occur when people feel personally responsible for their choice of action and the resulting consequences.

Large rewards or penalties that "over-justify" the target behavior can motivate people to perform safely for the wrong reasons. Under these circumstances, people are not likely to develop the kind of internal justification — or personal control — that sustains safe behavior in the absence of carrots and sticks.

Self-motivation can be decreased if a motivational program is seen as an attempt to control behavior. This underscores the importance of making sure praise, recognition and other behavior-based rewards are genuine.

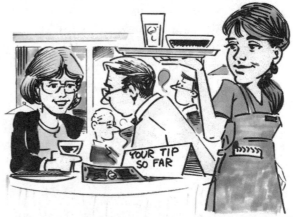

Behavior-based rewards and penalties make a difference.

Individuals or groups receiving special recognition must believe they truly earned the reward through their own efforts. When rewards are associated to one's own efforts, self-motivation increases because the person has a sense of being in control. Employees must see a connection between their own behavior and achievement of a patient-safety goal.

If given genuinely, interpersonal recognition, group celebration, and positive feedback improve internal, unobservable aspects of people. They make you feel better. This is a worthwhile outcome by itself. Plus, it's likely safety-related behaviors will be indirectly improved.

• Delivered appropriately, rewards always bring out the best in people because they improve those feelings states — self-esteem, self-efficacy, personal control, optimism, and belongingness — that improve quality of care. Look for opportunities to reward quality performance, and deliver the reward well.

12 How to facilitate self-directed behavior
Instilling a sense of personal responsibility

How do we go about changing consciously competent/other-directed behavior to consciously competent/self-directed behavior?

This is the best course of action for reducing risks and errors, because as we've discussed, other-directed behavior requires ongoing compliance mechanisms, and habits can put our brains into a mindless automatic mode, making it easy to slip up or forget a step.

What we're talking about here is facilitating a transition from safety accountability — "I'm working safely because someone is holding me accountable" — to safety responsibility — "I'm working safely because I'm holding myself accountable."

Here are five general recommendations, all based on behavioral research.[46]

1) Decrease top-down control for safety
Focus on fact-finding rather than fault-finding. Consider the disadvantages of punishment, and the differences between an unintended error and a calculated risk. Recognize how interpersonal and environmental context influences at-risk behavior.

2) Increase feelings of empowerment
Hold people accountable for safety performance numbers they can control. Set goals that are Specific, Motivational, Achievable, Relevant, and Trackable (SMART). Recognize progress and milestones toward successive accomplishments. Show genuine interest in others and increase the use of supportive interventions.

3) Help staff feel important
Increase opportunities for choice. Teach principles and guide the customization of procedures. Demonstrate the significance of proactive, People-Based Patient Safety™, and teach the value of emotional intelligence, including tech-

niques for communicating more effectively with others and yourself, using constructive self-talk. (See Chapter 4 on Thinking for research on the benefits of self-talk.)

4) Cultivate belonging and interpersonal trust

Improve interpersonal communication. Build group consensus for important decisions. Promote systems thinking and interdependence. Teach and demonstrate the principle of reciprocity — the fact that helping others activates a personal obligation to return the favor.

5) Teach and support safety self-management

Apply the Activator-Behavior-Consequence principle of behavioral safety to self-talk and self-management. Chapter 4 on Thinking covers this critical approach to developing safety responsibility and a culture of people actively caring for patient safety.

13 How to achieve compliance with safety rules
We use these techniques every day

Self-directed actions are most preferable, but there is no way around it — healthcare hierarchies and cultures often demand rules-driven, compliance-oriented behaviors. Social psychologists have researched techniques to strengthen compliance, and those most relevant to patient safety are reviewed here. Some might seem like common sense; that's because we use them every day.

1) Personal appeal

In general, people are most likely to comply with the wishes or instructions of someone they like. This is obvious, and points up the need for ingratiation (see bullet points below). Anyone seeking to get others to comply must ingratiate themselves to that group, at least to some extent. Indeed, this notion runs counter to the steep authority gradients common in healthcare. But if your goal is to bring individuals into compliance, social psychology research has verified a number

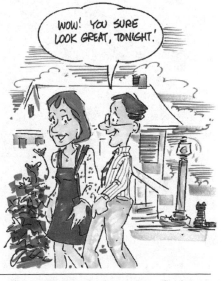

Ingratiation is common during "the dating game."

of common techniques to boost one's appeal to another person, or persons:[47]

• Demonstrate your agreement with the person or group on other matters before making the request;

• Offer genuine praise, recognition, or rewarding feedback;

• Use "name dropping" to show your association with people respected by the group you've targeted for compliance;

• Radiate positive nonverbal cues, such as smiles and friendly gestures, that show appreciation and interest in the people you want to reach.

The experience in healthcare is frequently the opposite of ingratiation. Compliance is too often defined by confrontation between an authoritative individual and a subordinate. Or a request to serve on a patient-safety steering committee or task force is presented in an impersonal memo or e-mail message. Although we understand this principle of ingratiation on a personal level, it's often not followed when making a request.

2) Start small

Social influence research demonstrates that someone who follows a small request is likely to comply with a larger request later. During the Korean War, Chinese communists used this technique on American prisoners by gradually escalating their demands that started with a few harmless requests. First, the prisoners were persuaded to speak or write trivial statements; then they were urged to copy or create statements that criticized American capitalism; eventually prisoners participated in group discussions of the advantages of communism, wrote self-criticisms, and gave public confessions of their wrong-doing.[48]

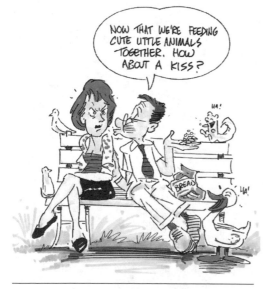

After a foot in the door, we expect more.

This "start small and build" strategy is successful in boosting product sales, monetary contributions to charities, and blood donations. In one study, researchers posed as volunteers in a local traffic safety campaign and went "cold calling" door-to-door to ask residents permission to install a large ugly sign in their front yards with the message "Drive Carefully." Only about 17 percent consented to this request. But 76 percent of residents who two weeks earlier had signed a safety legislation petition or had agreed to display a 3-inch square "Be a Safe Driver" sign in their home allowed the installation of the large sign.[49]

"Foot-in-the-door" techniques only work to increase safe behaviors when people comply with the initial small request. In fact, if the individual says "no" to the first request, this person might find it easier to refuse a subsequent, more important request. Thus, it might be important to build up your appeal (ingratiation) to ensure compliance with an initial small request. Or if circumstances suggest resistance could be forthcoming, you might consider using the next social influence technique — "door-in-the-face."

3) Shoot high

Here you start with an outrageous request. Something like, "Would you chair our patient-safety steering committee?" Then, when you receive the expected "no," you later make a smaller request — the one you wanted all along. This could be, "Would you participate in a patient-safety steering committee meeting?" Since

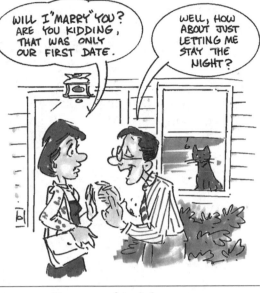

**Does a refusal deserve
a good turn?**

you showed willingness to "back down" from your initial request, subtle pressure is put on the person you want to influence to make a similar concession and agree this time. This exchange relates to the principle of reciprocity — another social psychology principle to consider when attempting to increase compliance with safe work practices.

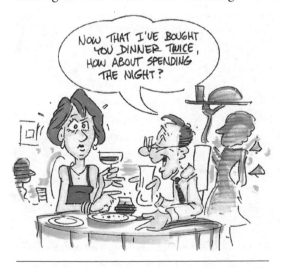

Does one good turn deserve another?

4) One good turn...

Some sociologists, anthropologists, and moral philosophers consider reciprocity a universal norm that motivates a good deal of interpersonal behavior.[50] Simply put, people are expected to help those who have helped them.

What does this mean for patient-safety rules compliance? Look for opportunities where, by following patient-safety rules, you make another person's job easier. Following infection control procedures reduces infection rates and makes everyone's job easier, and more rewarding. Keeping hallways clear allows everyone to move more freely.

Discuss in a group situations that relate to each of these social influence strategies. You will probably be able to identify past situations where these techniques were used intuitively without anyone realizing it. Or you might pick out certain situations that could have benefited from one or more of these tactics. Most importantly, however, you will be able to define specific ways to use these interpersonal influence techniques in the future to increase people's willingness to comply and get more involved in achieving a patient-safety culture.

Try to apply these principles whenever an opportunity occurs. You'll be setting an example, or modeling — another powerful social influence technique.

14 Two tools for promoting safety-related behaviors

Methods for focusing your thoughts and actions

Here are two tools to use before you take actions such as:
  • Administering medication
  • Hooking an intravenous tube
  • Answering a call button
  • Responding to a patient crashing
  • Handing off a patient
  • Beginning surgical procedures.

Critical behavior checklist

By now, you know how important it is to pay attention and stay fully aware of the task at hand. But in the chaotic healthcare environment, where distractions and interruptions go with the territory, how do we stay mindful of our behaviors? How do we remember all the steps and the many important details?

Before you start a procedure, pinpoint critical safe actions you need to take for patient safety, as well as potentially at-risk actions you need to avoid. Sometimes it's as simple as not touching a chart with a contaminated gloved hand. Sometimes, at-risk behavior is much more complicated. At other times, the safe behavior is more inconvenient or complicated.

This proactive process helps to ensure that, no matter how often a procedure is performed by a given practitioner, no step will be forgotten. It's often useful to write these critical actions on a "critical behavior checklist" for a particular task or procedure. Keep this checklist on hand before you begin the relevant task.

S.T.A.R.T. Checklist

The S.T.A.R.T. Checklist provides a simple way to remember to pinpoint critical actions before every procedure. It is best to jot down the specific steps as a prompt or reminder, rather than relying on memory.

STOP — Before every procedure, stop for one to two seconds to focus on the task at hand. This is how you focus your attention and consider all the steps needed for patient safety.

THINK — Define the critical safe actions you need to take. Consider the possible risk factors. For instance, is there a potential for dangerous drug interactions? What preventive actions are needed to keep the patient safe? What actions need to be avoided?

ACT — After developing a checklist of critical safe actions, you apply it to prompt the occurrence of safe behaviors and the avoidance of at-risk behaviors.

REVIEW — When the procedure is complete, revisit and evaluate the situation. Check for desired results.

TRACK — Finally, remember to follow up on the outcomes of your procedures. How is your patient feeling?

FAQ *Should employees be compensated for participating in patient-safety activities? What about education sessions or committees held off-hours?*

Healthcare employees should be compensated for their time in learning how to improve patient safety and in contributing their perspectives on how to improve patient safety. We are quick to invest in high-tech equipment, but do not always recognize the value of investing in people. At the same time, healthcare workers should be thrilled to learn new ways to reduce human error and improve patient safety. They should also be thrilled to contribute their wealth of experience to the development of interventions to improve patient safety.

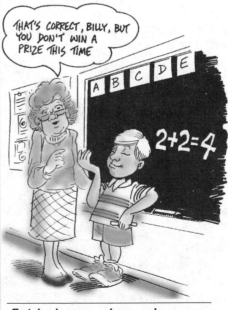

Extrinsic rewards can decrease intrinsic motivation and internal justification.

Psychologists have found that people want to be competent at what they believe is important. In other words, people want to be the best they can be when they are doing important stuff. Healthcare workers perform critically important work, and want to be the best they can be at helping their patients. So if healthcare workers believe patient-safety seminars and focus groups will improve their competency at doing their important work, they will surely participate even if the compensation is not great.

FAQ *How do you put an end to unacceptable behavior — intentional violation of known rules or abusive, bullying behavior?*

Corrective coaching is the quick answer. Address the problem in specific behavioral terms with the individual who needs to improve, explore ways to make the improvement including interpersonal support needed, and obtain a personal commitment to improve. This is the essence of "positive discipline."[51]

Corrective coaching should be used in place of punishment. But there are times when individuals intentionally disregard rules or do not have the necessary motivation to maintain competence. In these cases, discipline supports cultural values.

But before forcing a person off the bus, it is important and ethical to implement corrective coaching so the individual has the opportunity to improve:

• First, the person needs to identify and own up to the inappropriate behavior.

• Then the individual needs to explore ways to improve, often with the help of other staff.

• After identifying a plan of action for improvement, the person needs to make a commitment to act.

• Subsequent observations from other staff should verify improvement in terms of observable behaviors.

If any of these steps do not occur, the corrective action is not complete and will probably fail.

How many chances do we give an individual to fail? That depends on many factors, including the individual's genuine willingness to try again, and the risk to patient welfare. Without the motivation to improve or the appropriate competence, it is best to remove the individual from their position. As indicated above, this is beneficial to everyone involved.

CHAPTER 3 *Coaching*

In this chapter you'll learn:

1 Everyone is a coach
Coaches model what they teach and advocate

Coaching for People-Based Patient Safety™ focuses on how to prevent human error through one-on-one conversations and teamwork.

Let's get right to the heart of the matter: the true value of safety coaching comes not through the information we collect or disseminate. It's in the conversation — the dialogue we have with each other about what we observe and think about (recall Chapter 2 on Acting).

The human dynamics of patient safety are more complex than training handouts and mere checks on a behavioral checklist. Checklists in fact can limit development of self-accountability and can have only short-term benefits — reflected in the common "pencil-whipping" label given to some applications of behavioral checklists.

"Checklists can't be your only change-agent for patient safety," says a physician and patient-safety coleader at a children's hospital. "People will tune out a preponderance of checklists. They'll just say, 'I know how to do this.'"

People-Based Patient Safety™ (PBPS) takes your prevention efforts beyond "checklist medicine." Everyone coaches for safety: nurses, physicians, pharmacists, lab techs, transporters, department heads and administrators — the entire organization.

Why should everyone coach?

Because coaching develops the self-directed accountability needed for a sustained, long-term commitment to safety. Coaches feel obligated to adopt principles and procedures they teach and advocate. To be sure, it might be prudent to start a PBPS coaching process with a select number of staff — those who've shown an interest or concern for patient safety. It depends on your organization's culture, especially the level of interdependency and interpersonal trust that exists. But it's expected that eventually all employees will coach each other to prevent medical errors and patient harm.

In this chapter we discuss both "formal" and "informal" coaching. Formal coaching parallels standard observation and feedback sessions, which employ a checklist of critical behaviors, and have met with documented success in reducing nosocomial infection rates. Informal coaching involves brief personal conversations to maintain daily attention — situational awareness — to safe versus risky behaviors and conditions.

By focusing on ongoing interpersonal communication more than checklists and training lectures you increase both the frequency and quality of informal coaching. And this leads to self-coaching, which is essential for the many front-line caregivers working alone.

Expert Q&A   Coaching on the frontlines

Lori A. Paine, RN, MS, is the patient-safety coordinator for The Johns Hopkins Hospital.

Q *You were the first person hired into Hopkins' Center for Innovation in Quality Patient Care, as a coach overseeing the "Touch Time" initiative. The objective was to find ways to increase the time nurses spend at bedside. What makes for a good patient-safety coach?*

A *As a coach you can't own patient safety, you can't write the prescription. You're there to help, to give support, educate and to advise. To do that, you have to get buy-in from local unit leadership first. You can't go in as a know-it-all.*

With Touch Time, we saw coaching as a way to use the intellectual capital of our people. We have a lot of people here with expertise, who know what the solutions can be. We needed to resource our frontline people with support to collect data and analyze the roots of problems. With Touch Time, we wanted to get nurses back to the core of their business. We wanted to find ways for nurses to make better use of their time.

One thing is to address concerns or skepticism up-front. There was the fear the Touch Time initiative was like some of those re-engineering ideas in the '90s, where quality was used as a cover for cost-cutting. That the checkbook, not the patient, was driving it.

I worked with volunteer units, asking nurses what their needs were. Where were the bottlenecks, where were they wasting time? Frontline people told us they didn't have the time, skills or understanding of methods to make improvements, to increase bedside Touch Time. So we pulled a team together to study time-and-motion data, to learn why nurses were pulled away from bedside. Some solutions had to do with better communication: using two-way pagers and fax machines with doctors and pharmacists.

2 Coaching is conversing

"Healthcare is fundamentally about relationships, patients with doctors, doctors to doctors, department to department." — Rosemary Gibson, senior project officer, Robert Wood Johnson Foundation, and author, *Wall of Silence.*

"Much of what passes for communication in healthcare is superficial. Talking about patient safety makes many people uncomfortable. There's a fear of litigation,

and undermining public confidence. Healthcare is really dangerous. How are we going to talk honestly about its risks?" — Martin Hatlie, president, Partnership for Patient Safety.

Conversations rule

Did you ever think your efforts to keep patients from harm and prevent errors throughout your system are determined more by everyday conversation than anything else?

We're convinced the way we talk to ourselves (intrapersonal communication) and to others (interpersonal communication) is a powerful, pervasive determinant of safety excellence. In industry we've seen the dramatic success companies experience with behavioral safety is essentially due to an increase in the quality and quantity of interpersonal conversation about safety. This ripple effect throughout an organization in turn improves intrapersonal conversations, bolstering one's sense of personal control and optimism regarding their ability to prevent slips and mistakes and protect patients from harm.

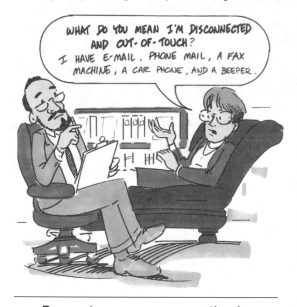

Person-to-person conversation has no substitute.

We'd like to convince you of the power of conversation to penetrate a culture and plant seeds of change. We believe you won't spend the time and effort to hone your coaching skills until you truly appreciate the clout that conversation carries.

Consider these stories:

• To break through hierarchical barriers and mobilize its workforce around patient safety, a hospital treats a group of physicians and nurses to a pleasant, quiet dinner off-site. They're asked to consider this question: How can the hospital support collaboration between doctors and nurses and make the facility safer? This leads to a realistic and relaxed conversation that produces a number of ideas for more reliable ways of working as a team.

• The Safest in America coalition in the Minneapolis/St. Paul area brings together CEOs representing 10 area healthcare systems and 27 hospitals, plus the Mayo Clinic in Rochester, Minnesota, for quarterly meetings to reach agreement on patient-safety protocols to be used by the participants.

"Reaching a consensus is very difficult on a number of initiatives because everyone believes their practices are already good. No one says, 'We're sloppy and lousy,'" reports David Page, chairman of the coalition and CEO of

Fairview Health Services. "It's like building a fire with wet wood. You have to protect it and fan it and build it slowly." Some organizations will grumble, he says, but if the majority create a standard of practice, others come aboard out of a sense of shared mission, good will, or possible legal ramifications, he says. The coalition has hammered out directives for writing prescriptions and surgery site markings and has work groups addressing rapid response teams and hospital-acquired infections.

• At The Johns Hopkins Hospital, units volunteering to adopt the Comprehensive Unit-based Safety Program (CUSP) start by answering this question: How is the next patient in this unit going to be harmed, and what can be done to prevent that harm? "Frontline personnel need to be allowed to express their concerns," says Hopkins' patient-safety coordinator Lori Paine. "Staff knows the problems and solutions. There are a lot of people here with expertise."

Culture is conversation

Perhaps it's fair to say culture is conversation — both spoken and unspoken. Absence of conversation can initiate or permit resentment, frustration and conflict to fester. Silence sinks morale and productivity, and stifles the willingness to take on new initiatives like patient safety. On the other hand, the occurrence of conversation — authentic, direct talk — can chip away at walls and silos and breathe fresh air into an organization. "Let's talk it out," as the saying goes, with the emphasis on getting safety issues and risks out in the open.

Here's how the quality of conversation can make or break working relationships — and whole cultures:

• We define the support, loyalty and courage of our bosses and our coworkers by the way we talk about them, both to ourselves and to others. Our mental scripts and verbal behaviors are powerful — giving meaning to the values that define our connections to other people, and to organizations. When groups communicate to discuss and define these values (respect versus disrespect, openness versus secrecy, and so on) we develop a culture.

• This development process can occur in unspoken ways. Think of the customs or unwritten rules we heed without mention:

The boss doesn't want to hear about a close call....

High seniority carries unspoken privileges — favoritism — which is certainly not expressed....

A department knows the unspoken characteristics that bias their managers' performance appraisals, from gender and personality to cocktails after work.

• Public discourse also helps mold an organization's culture by defining its public image. Some healthcare systems are lauded and awarded for their patient-safety endeavors, which helps reputations and even market-branding; others are lacerated in the press for errors and mistakes that have harmed patients, setting the stage for reactive or punitive cultural reforms.

• The way people talk affects not only cultural images and brand

Talking Points

Conversations we have with ourselves and others have the power to:

• *Initiate or fuel conflict*

• *Defuse or eliminate conflict*

• *Build self-esteem*

• *Shape public image*

• *Increase or decrease safety motivation*

• *Shape an organization's safety image*

• *Define work cultures, including patient-safety cultures*

• *"Air out" — or ventilate differences of opinion — to provide the oxygen needed for organic growth of initiatives*

• *Raise or lower patient throughput (productivity)*

• *Improve or hinder safety performance*

• *Achieve safety breakthroughs.*

reputations, but personal self-image or self-esteem. We can focus our self-talk on the good things people say about us, or on critical statements we've heard about us. The result is a certain kind of self-talk we call "interpretation." Such intrapersonal communication can raise or lower the way we feel about ourselves. In other words, our self-esteem can go up or down according to how we talk to ourselves about the way others talk about us.

• Want to make a breakthrough in patient safety? In his provocative book *Leadership & the Art of Conversation,*[1] Kim Krisco defines a breakthrough as going beyond business-as-usual and getting more than expected. This requires people to realize new possibilities, commit to going for more, and then make a concerted effort to overcome barriers. How is this done? You guessed it — through conversation.

Expect resistance to change, warns Krisco. The greater the change, the greater the resistance. But remember, most barriers are interpretations or people's self-talk about what is happening in an organization. Conversation, both interpersonal and intrapersonal, enables us to shine light on negative interpretations, hold them up for examination, weigh the advantages of possible alternatives, and then replace old views with new expectations.

The status of patient safety in your organization is largely determined by how it is talked about, from the boardroom to the supply room. Whether we feel responsible for preventing harm to patients and commit to go for a break-through depends on our interpretation of the safety-related conversations we hear. Are we listening to shallow spin about the need for patient safety — mere lip service — or are we hearing serious, succinct dialog about finding and fixing the causes of preventable harm?

③ Seven strategies to improve conversations about safety
Conversations are a leading indicator of involvement

Given the power of conversation to resolve conflict; achieve breakthrough; and define image, self-esteem, and culture, we obviously need to direct this powerful tool to improve patient safety. How do we maximize interpersonal and intrapersonal conversations? What kinds of conversations are more likely to stimulate and maintain improvements?

Consider these seven strategies for improving safety-related conversations between people. Each one can get staff more involved in safety, and improve your overall level of patient-safety performance.

1) Don't look back

Let's begin by considering how frequently conversations play-back past events, especially negative experiences. We know this from personal experience and from watching the nightly news. Regarding risk prevention in healthcare, sentinel and adverse event root-cause analyses are discussions about past failures. They are of course necessary exercises, but they cannot be the only forums for discussing issues relating to patient safety. To improve protective measures, we need to move conversations — both our "self-talk" and conversations with others — from recounting the past to focusing on future possibilities. From there we can develop suitable action plans.

So how do you pull this off? Say you approach someone about getting more involved in a patient-safety initiative and they reply, "I filed an incident report last year and never heard a word about it." Where do you take the conversation from here?

This is really a matter of leadership, as discussed in Kim Krisco's book. Leaders help people move their conversations from the past to the future and then back to the present (where you begin the development of a relevant corrective action plan). To direct the flow of a conversation in this way, you first must recognize and appreciate what the other person has to say. Then shift the focus toward the future. Remember, you're approaching this person to discuss possibilities for safety improvement and specific ways to get started now.

(For more on how to handle safety-related complaints, see Section 9 later in this chapter on "Responding to Resistance.")

2) Seek commitment

Your objective in this kind of conversation is to get a commitment from the other person. Safety-related conversations are productive when someone commits to taking a specific action — it could be getting behind an incident reporting effort, completing a culture survey on patient safety, or discussing a near-harm experience in a unit meeting.

A verbal commitment also tells you something is happening on an intrapersonal level, within that other person. It's a sign the person is becoming motivated. Then you can proceed to talk about how that commitment can be supported, or how to hold the individual accountable.

3) Stop and listen

Be careful when you try to influence the behavior of others. Sometimes a passion for safety can lead to an overly directive approach. You know from personal experience, and clinical psychologists have shown, it's better to give advice in a nondirective manner, especially over the long term.

Think about it: How do you respond when someone bluntly tells you what to do? You might follow the instruction, especially if it comes from someone with the power to control your consequences. But will you be motivated to make a permanent change?

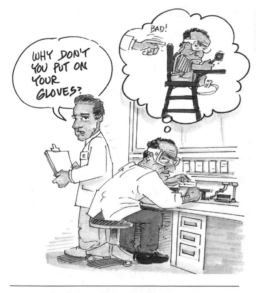

Safety directives can be perceived as confrontations.

"For God's sake don't get command and control on people," says the CEO of one Midwest hospital. "Command and control comes out as a patient-safety edict. Get too pushy and adamant and people feel like they're getting punished."

Exactly. Conversations that come off as "adult-child" confrontations often fall apart. Sure you mean well, but other people might not see it that way. Play it "safe." Try to be more nondirective.

Nondirective psychotherapy revolves around active listening. The objective is to get clients to reveal their concerns, problems, and solutions on their own terms. The therapist's role is to be a passive catalyst, enabling and facilitating a conversation directed and owned by the client. Not that safety coaches should become therapists, but we can take some useful lessons from this nondirective approach.[2] This surely applies to efforts involved in getting patients to take a more active role in their own health, and safety. (See Section 10 in this chapter on "Coaching Patients.")

Immerse yourself in the conversation. "You have to listen, really listen, to the content of complaints," relating to patient safety, says Martin Hatlie, president, Partnership for Patient Safety. He calls it "active, immersed listening."

4) Ask questions first

Instead of telling people what to do, try this: Get them to tell you, in their own words, what they ought to be doing to reduce risk. You can do this by asking questions with a sincere and caring demeanor. Avoid at all costs a sarcastic or demeaning tone.

First, compliment any safe behaviors you noticed. It could be something as simple as handwashing or taking the time to use two patient identifiers before drawing blood, or as bold as disclosing an error or calling for a rapid response team. It's important to emphasize positives because so much of patient-safety education and training revolves around negative stories, failures, things gone wrong.

"Focus on what's being done well," says Hatlie. "Talking about problems all the time pulls down the energy of an organization."

Then move on to the seemingly at-risk behavior by asking something like, "Is there a safer way to transfer patient information at the end of the shift? We seem awfully rushed." You might, in fact, find your presumptions to be imperfect, in this case about hand-offs. The "expert" on the job might know something you don't.

By asking questions you're always going to learn something. If nothing else, you'll hear the rationale behind taking a risk over choosing the safer alternative. You might uncover a barrier to safety you can then help the person overcome.

Remember, it's only natural to offer a defense for taking a risk. It's a matter of protecting one's self-esteem. Let it pass. Remind yourself when someone owns up to his or her mistake — even under a cloud of excuses — your nondirective approach is beginning to draw the person out and bring about the change you desire.

5) Use words wisely

But what if the person doesn't give a satisfactory answer to your question about safer alternatives? What if the individual doesn't seem to know your SBAR or read-back protocols? That's when you need to shift the conversation from nondirective to directive. You need to give behavior-focused advice. "Remember, SBAR is our Situation-Background-Assessment-Recommendation procedure for briefings on a patient's condition. Let's go over it."

In this case, you might start with the phrase, "As you know." Safety consultant John Drebinger advises always to use this as an opener.[3] Launch the

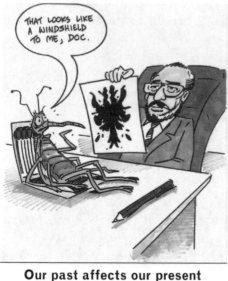

Our past affects our present thinking.

conversation with a phrase that implies the person really does know the safe way to perform, but for some reason just overlooked it (or forgot) this time. This could happen to anyone. Such an opening can help prevent others from feeling their intelligence or safety knowledge has been insulted.

6) Beware of bias

Every conversation you have with someone is biased. You can't get around it. From personal experience, people develop opinions and attitudes that filter the words we hear, the way we interpret those words, and what we say in response. Every conversation influences how we process and interpret the next conversation.

Personal biases cause people to filter you out. By asking for their input upfront, you reduce the likelihood they will later tune you out. It's the principle of reciprocity: By listening first, you increase the odds the other person will do likewise, and listen to you.

Don't allow your prejudices about a speaker color or restrict what you hear. Do you ever listen less closely to certain individuals, perhaps because the person seldom has anything useful to say or because you think you can predict what they'll say? Tell yourself you're not listening to someone, rather you're listening for something. "Content," Hatlie calls it. You're not listening reactively to confirm a prejudice — you're listening in a probing way for content — clues or possibilities to solve a safety issue.

Pay close attention to body language and tone in conversations. Method of delivery can reveal as much, or more, information as the words themselves. Listen for passion, commitment, and caring. If nothing else, you can learn whether the messenger understands and believes the message. And perhaps you'll learn a new method for delivering a message yourself.

7) Plant words to improve self-image

Want to change how others perceive you? Change the conversations people are having about you.

Here's what we mean: Perhaps you suspect colleagues consider you a "safety-control freak." You know, someone who flips out over small individual transgressions, with no thought for system pressures everyone works under. Well, you might mention to your colleagues that after reviewing incident reports and asking around you see how even good people can screw up in a faulty system. Of course you need to actually practice these techniques. If you focus on new positive qualities rather than past inadequacies in your conversations with others and with yourself, you're on your way to rehabilitating your self-image and self-esteem.

Conversation checklist
To get the most from safety-related conversations:
- *Show genuine interest.*
- *Listen attentively.*
- *Emphasize positive actions you've observed.*
- *Draw out responses from the other person.*
- *Get them to tell you what should be done to be sufficiently safe.*
- *Ask questions with a sincere and caring demeanor.*
- *Act as if you don't know the answer, even though you think you do.*
- *Shift the focus to future ways of improving safety.*
- *Bring the conversation from future to present by focusing on what can be done now to improve.*
- *Seek a verbal commitment to embrace a desirable corrective action plan.*

4 How to give coaching feedback
A critical component of coaching conversations

How do you use interpersonal feedback to improve patient safety? Here you'll find a list of 20 guidelines to help you deliver feedback effectively. It's a critical tool for influencing the type of safe behavior you want to see on the floor, in a department, during slow times or crises, any situation where actions affect patient welfare.

1. Feedback can be positive or negative, and can influence the quality and frequency of performance.

2. When you want to motivate the frequency of a particular behavior, try to deliver appropriate feedback as soon after the target behavior as feasible.

3. Safe behavior should be followed by positive feedback (or praise) to support that behavior and increase the odds it will occur again.

4. At-risk behavior should be interrupted immediately with corrective feedback to stop the behavior and prevent harm.

5. When you see an at-risk behavior, you should usually do more than just attempt to stop it. If possible, give specific direction for making the behavior more safe. Use your judgment here; your reaction depends on circumstances.

6. Take note of the corrective action needed to make a certain behavior safer, and when an occasion arises for that behavior to occur again, offer instruction at this time — as an activator.

7. Sometimes at-risk behaviors begin and end too quickly during crisis situations for you to offer any sort of feedback. But of course you need to review what happened to prevent future risks. We're not talking about failure events and morbidity and mortality (M&M) conferences, but more informal coaching feedback sessions. And if you observe a sequence of at-risk behaviors, corrective feedback following one behavior will serve to direct the next behavior.

8. If the opportunity for another possible at-risk behavior is delayed — perhaps it's a matter of improper patient lifting — feedback is more powerful if given later, preceding an opportunity to be safe or at-risk. Wait until you see another patient being lifted. Delaying such correction is also less embarrassing for the performer.

9. It's not necessary for you to tell the person about the prior at-risk observation, just remind him or her to perform the upcoming behavior in a safe manner. Then, statements like "Remember to double-check identifiers" and "Don't forget to ask questions" come across as friendly and caring reminders rather than "gotcha" indictments.

10. Always remember as a coach, your feedback needs to focus on specific safe or at-risk behavior.

11. Feedback needs to be straightforward and objective. Ambiguous or subjective language that attempts to judge internal states of mind is not useful, and can be counterproductive. For example, a statement like, "What in the world were you thinking?" only adds resentment and lessens acceptance of your message.

12. When you give positive statements watch for the use of "but" — an instant deflator. Rather than giving pure praise or appreciation, we often feel obligated to add a negative (or corrective feedback) statement to balance the communication. Such a mixed message can weaken your feedback. Some people hear only the positive; some hear only the negative; and others discount both messages.

13. It's often best to narrow the focus of your feedback. Rather than combining both positive and negative feedback in one exchange or overloading a person with several behaviors to improve, direct your advice to one area of performance.

14. It's much better to give people concise feedback messages consistently over weeks or months than to give people fewer but longer feedback debriefings that often mix potentially confusing motivators and directives. Keep it simple.

15. Motivational feedback to increase or decrease the frequency of behavior should follow the target behavior as soon as possible. On the other hand, when the purpose of behavioral feedback is to shape the quality of a response, it often makes sense to give such direction as an activator (preceding the next opportunity to perform the target behavior).

Remember, the activator-behavior-consequence model of behavior change reflects the basic principle that behavior (B) is directed by activators (A) and motivated by consequences (C). Activators precede our actions and are most apt to influence the quality of our performance (how we do things); consequences usually influence the quantity of our performance (how often we do things).

16. Receiving feedback about errors can be perceived as punishing and frustrating if the performer doesn't have the chance to correct the observed errors in the near future. When the person eventually receives that chance to correct the behavior, the advice might be forgotten. By giving corrective feedback as close as possible to the next opportunity for the behavior to recur, you increase its directive influence. And you reduce the potential negative effect of catching a person making a mistake without giving him the opportunity to "redeem" himself.

17. Feedback should fit the situation. Specific and well-timed feedback must be appropriate for the needs, abilities, and expectations of the person on the receiving end. It should be expressed in language the performer can understand and appreciate, and it should be customized for the performer's abilities at the particular task.

When people are learning a task, directive feedback needs to be detailed and perhaps accompanied with a behavioral demonstration. In such learning situations, it's important to match the advice with the performer's achievement level. Don't give more advice than the individual can grasp in one feedback session.

Often at-risk behavior is performed by experienced staff. They know how to do the job safely, but they have developed poor habits or are just taking a risky short-cut. It could be insulting and

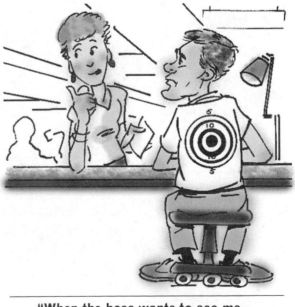

**"When the boss wants to see me,
I expect the worst."**

demeaning to give professionals detailed instructions about the safe way to complete their job. In these situations, it's appropriate to give brief corrective feedback as a reminder to be safe and model the right example for others.

18. Giving good feedback requires up-to-date knowledge of the performer's abilities regarding a certain task. It also requires specific knowledge about the safe and at-risk ways of performing the task. This is a prime reason why the most effective safety coaching usually occurs between peers on the same team.

19. Feedback will be ineffective if it's viewed as bullying or an intimidating show of authority or expertise. Remember, the only reason for giving patient-safety-related feedback is to prevent harm to patients.

20. The "gotcha" perspective associated with safety feedback often blunts a manager's sincere attempt to correct at-risk behavior. Corrective feedback is often perceived as most genuine or "real" when it occurs between coworkers on the same team or in the same unit. These individuals know more about the situation and the people involved, and thus have sufficient information and opportunity to give the best feedback.

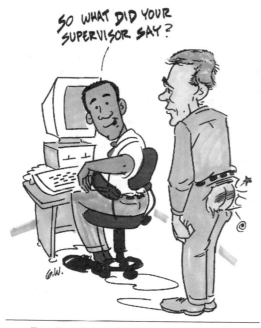

Feedback is often more negative than positive.

These 20 guidelines can be summarized by the word "SOAR." Effective feedback delivery must be Specific, On time, Appropriate, and Real.

We think it's important to reiterate the special value in peers giving each other safety-related feedback. Coworkers' comments are less likely to come across as a "gotcha" indictment of inferior performance, and more in the spirit of "we're in this together" to be the best we can be. Plus, peers are more likely to be "right there" when immediate feedback is necessary. And they can best shape a message — probably without even giving it much thought — to the expectations, abilities, and experience level of the recipient. Finally, encouragement — or especially corrections from a coworker — are more apt to be taken as a sign of true caring.

5 Coaching characteristics

Spell it out: Care – Observe – Analyze – Communicate – Help

The five letters of the word COACH can be used as a mnemonic to remember the basic characteristics of effective coaching — Care, Observe, Analyze, Communicate and Help.

"C" for Care

Effective coaching requires basic communication skills, as we've noted, including active listening and persuasive speaking. Role-playing exercises on how to deliver and receive behavioral feedback are invaluable to develop effective coaching skills.

Coaching training should illustrate the need to separate behavior (actions) from person factors (attitudes and feelings). This is how you enable corrective feedback to target behaviors without "stepping on" feelings.

For example, people need to understand "human nature is prone to human lapses," as one physician puts it (as in unconscious incompetence). Behavior-specific feedback is required for skill-building. Thus, corrective feedback revealing at-risk behavior will be appreciated when given correctly. But it must start with the understanding that "a person can do everything right and still harm someone," as a nurse told us.

We want to emphasize "when given correctly." Your feedback should be specific (with regard to a particular behavior) and timely (delivered soon after the behavior occurs). If possible, it should be given in a private, one-on-one situation to avoid potential interference or embarrassment from others.

Certainly, you can't pull a nurse from the OR for a brief feedback session. Some one-on-one conversations might have to wait for a trip to the cafeteria or a walk to another department. At other times, however, there can be no waiting at all — intervention must be immediate when possible harm to a patient is imminent.

A safety coach must actively listen with appropriate body language and verbal responses when an employee on the receiving end of feedback reacts to comments. This is how you show sincere concern for the feelings and commitment of the person receiving feedback. The best listeners show they are paying attention with facial cues and posture. They ask for more details ("Tell me more"), accept feelings as stated without interpretation, and avoid self-centered statements that can stifle disclosure ("When I worked in your department, I always checked every infusion pump").

"As a coach, you can never go in with a know-it-all prescription," says Lori Paine, patient-safety coordinator for The Johns Hopkins Hospital.

Expert Q&A   *What is a healing relationship?*

Lori Nichols is director of the Whatcom Health Information Network and director of the Pursuing Perfection Program in Whatcom County, Bellingham, Washington.

Q *The patient-centered care model of your Pursuing Perfection Program employs specially trained clinical care specialists to counsel patients. They navigate and translate the healthcare system for patients, act as a coach and sometimes literally a lifeguard. The objective is to help patients self-manage daily treatment of chronic illnesses. "Loving competence" and "healing relationships" are integral to this process. What is a "healing relationship"?*

A *The healing relationship is a continuous relationship, not necessarily a curing relationship. It's approaching the patient as a whole person, not the heart failure in Room 4. It's taking time to get to know the individual, learning from the individual, and having conversations around that.*

When you break an ankle, the healthcare system is good at fixing the problem. Chronic disease requires more continuous care and involvement. Loving competence is understanding and respecting where the patient is: what's important to that individual, knowing and addressing how they learn, what special concerns they have, what barriers get in the way of them following the doctor's advice.

These relationships don't exist due to constraints of the current system. Healthcare used to be more personal. It has evolved into a production model with more time intrusions on caregivers, more paperwork, misaligned reimbursement incentives. The system is very broken. Providing translators, navigators and negotiators to look after and work with patients is essential now — we didn't need it before.

"O" for Observe

Safety coaches observe objectively and systematically. They look for both safe and at-risk behavior. Actions that "go beyond the call of duty" for the safety of a patient should especially be noted.

As a coach, you must know exactly what behavior is desired and undesired. This is where developing a checklist of safe and at-risk behaviors can be beneficial. At Sentara Healthcare System in Virginia, a team of 25 employees and 14 physicians drew up a set of behavior-based expectations through brainstorming sessions and identifying the casual factors in a score of significant events. Among the short list of expectations, every Sentara employee is expected to take a quick one- or two-second pause for a mental run-through before starting a job or procedure, and practice the "5 Ps" of a competent hand-off — reviewing the Patient, Problem, Purpose, Procedures and Precautions.

"A" for Analyze

After observation comes interpretation. Coaches need to explore why certain behaviors are occurring.

You'll recall from the previous chapter on Acting that certain at-risk behaviors occur because they are directed by activators, such as patient volume, at-risk examples set by peers, and inconsistent or mixed messages from management. And, at-risk behaviors are often motivated by one or more consequences (comfort, time-savings, and mentor or peer approval). This is the activator-behavior-consequence model that shapes behavior.

Remember, as a safety coach, you can be both an activator and a motivator. The way you observe, analyze, and communicate can activate safe behaviors through instructions, reminders, individual and group discussions. And you can motivate repeated safe behavior through verbal feedback, individual recognition, and group celebrations.

"C" for Communicate

Interpersonal communication is the critical intervention step of safety coaching. Everyone wants to take steps to improve patient safety and prevent risks, but at the same time many people resist giving and receiving the kind of communication that facilitates beneficial change. The "same old routine" is familiar, non-threatening, secure, and relatively easy. Change-focused communication can threaten one's sense of independence and authority.

Some people perceive feedback that implies personal change as an indictment of their work style, competence, or dedication. This reaction is most likely to occur when someone is being asked to change dramatically, and when current risky procedures have been ingrained for years.

To overcome defiance or denial, skip dramatic confrontations. Steer clear of disruptive confrontation — remember we're talking about coaching here, not bossing people around. And emphasize incremental "fine tuning." Don't overreach. You can't turn around the *Titanic* in a day, says Lori Paine.

Look for opportunities to recognize or support "small win" patient-safety improvements on your floor or in your department. Obviously, at-risk behavior needs to be corrected, but effective coaches realize people do not like to be criticized and are apt to reject or deny a negative communication about the need to change.

Before suggesting a need for specific change, attempt to communicate in a positive (or at least neutral) way by finding something positive to say about the situation (if only to state sincere concern for the safety of patients in a unit).

"H" for Help

Actually, "help" summarizes the mission of a patient-safety coach. The goal is to help healthcare workers prevent unintentional harm to patients. The key is to get people to accept feedback. We use the letters in the word HELP as reminders:

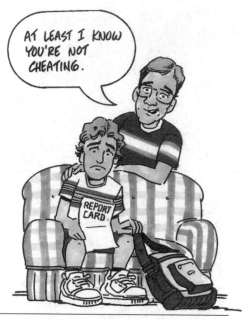

Look for the silver lining to build self-esteem.

"H" for humor. Safety is certainly serious business, but sometimes a little humor can increase interest and decrease resistance. It can help diffuse a stressful situation.

"E" for esteem. People who feel diminished or demeaned by criticism are not likely to go beyond the call of duty for a patient's welfare. Choose your words carefully (emphasizing the positive over the negative) in an attempt to build or avoid lessening another person's sense of self-worth and personal control.

"L" for listen. One of the most powerful and convenient ways to build trust is to listen attentively to another person. The person can interpret this active listening as a reflection of appreciation. After a coach actively listens, his or her message is more likely to be heard and accepted.

Peter Perreiah coaches hospital staff for the Pittsburgh Regional Healthcare Initiative, and he builds trust and confidence in his intentions by first listening to complaints. "Tell us what is wasting your time," he asks staff. He looks for small-win fixes, moves on from quality to safety issues, and gradually "opens eyes and starts making believers" in what can be accomplished in preventing errors and improving patient care.

"P" for praise. Praising another person, or a group or team, for a specific accomplishment is a powerful way to build trust and confidence. If the praise is genuine and targets a particular behavior — handwashing, gloving, speaking up, reporting, reading back, you name it — the odds of the behavior occurring again increase. This is the basic principle of positive reinforcement. It motivates people to continue their safe behaviors and to look for ways to reduce errors and prevent harm to patients.

6 Recognizing positive actions for patient safety

Satisfy a craving in us all

William James, the first great American psychologist, wrote "the deepest principle in human nature is the craving to be appreciated."[4] Giving and receiving recognition well is how we satisfy this hunger. Plus, we don't think there's a better way to cultivate an organizational culture that truly embraces patient safety and error prevention.

How many times have you heard: "We can't learn unless we make mistakes"? This might make us feel better about the errors of our ways, but nothing could be further from the truth in healthcare, where mistakes can be fatal. Moreover, behavioral scientists have shown convincingly that success — not failure — produces optimal learning.[5]

A negative consequence — blame or punishment — following a mistake only tells us what *not* to do. It provides no specific direction for problem-solving. And overemphasizing a mistake can discourage us from continuing the learning process. This is the risk of current media brow-beating over patient errors and tragedies.

In recent years we've witnessed an abundance of stinging press coverage about tragedies due to errors in patient care; meanwhile the positive consequences of effective patient care are unobserved and essentially ignored. Thus, if we want people to recognize the positive consequences in patient care, we need to do things to make them salient.

The personal story of an error that led to a negative outcome is certainly attention-getting and facilitates a "failure-avoidance" mindset. This tactic is important because it makes patient safety personal and emotional. But it's necessary to follow the personal story with the specific goal-directed actions needed to prevent errors and negative consequences. The focus must change to achievement.

In other words, healthcare workers need individual recognition and group celebrations for their progress and achievements in the realm of patient safety.

Consider the "patient-safety share." Start group discussions or team meetings with the simple question: "Does anybody have a patient-safety share?" Of course, people won't understand the question without an initial explanation. The patient-safety share merely asks people to disclose something they have done recently for patient safety. We're talking small wins. Helping a colleague out of a jam. Filing a safety suggestion. Catching a mislabeled specimen. Cleaning up someone else's spill in a hallway. This is a good way to break the ice and kick off a meeting on a positive, achievement-oriented note.

The results of a patient safety-share process can be remarkable, based on evidence we've seen in industry. People will start talking and thinking about a range of possible actions for patient safety. When they hear others report a safety-share experience, they'll learn things they can do and recall behaviors they performed for patient safety. It can bring patient safety down to a local level, and spark a shift from "failure-avoidance" to "success seeking."

Our vision for a robust Patient-Safety Culture is zero negative events, but our goals are set on a series of achievements needed to reach this vision. So we balance failure avoiding and success seeking. The safety share puts the daily focus on success seeking, with an ultimate purpose of avoiding failure.

Seven guidelines

If you decide to give positive "safety shares" a try, here are seven guidelines for presenting quality recognition:

Be on time

People need to know what they did to earn your appreciation. Then they are motivated to continue that behavior. So timely feedback is important. If it's necessary to delay recognition, when you do give it relive the behavior or activities that were noteworthy. Talk specifically about the performance. Don't hesitate to ask the recipient to recall aspects of the situation and the desirable behavior.

Get personal

Recognition should not be generic. There's no such thing as "one size fits all" recognition.

It's tempting to say "we appreciate" rather than "I appreciate," and to refer to organizational gratitude rather than personal acknowledgment. But speaking for the hospital or clinic or group practice or whatever can come across as impersonal and rhetorical. Of course it's appropriate to reflect the values of the organization when giving recognition, but the focus should be personal.

Take it to a higher level

Adding a universal value like leadership, integrity, trustworthiness, or actively caring to your recognition statement obviously makes what you're saying more rewarding. This acknowledges a higher-order quality, a potent way to boost self-esteem and make recognition more memorable. But it's important to state the specific behavior first, and then make an obvious linkage between the behavior and the positive value it reflects.

Go one-on-one

It's customary to recognize individuals in front of a group. Just think of any awards banquet. Many coaches and leaders take the lead from sporting events and give individual recognition in group settings. But some people feel embarrassed when singled out in front of a group. There might be accusations of "sucking up."

Be careful when giving public praise. Recognizing a person in public can be seen as favoritism by individuals who feel they did equally well, but did not get praised. Don't set up any sort of ranking that could create a win/lose atmosphere — perhaps appropriate for sporting events but not in healthcare settings where everyone needs to be on board for patient safety.

Recognizing teams of workers can be done in a group setting. Since individual responsibility is diffused or dispersed across the team, there's minimal risk of individual embarrassment or peer harassment.

Remember, though, team achievement rarely results from equal performances by all team members. It's important to deliver private recognition to those who went beyond the call of duty for the sake of their team.

Let it sink in

Healthcare is an especially fast-track and many times chaotic world. Often you need to communicate as much information as possible when you finally get in touch with a busy person. So after recognizing a person's special efforts for patient safety, we might be tempted to tag on a bunch of unrelated statements, even a request for additional behavior. This comes across as "I appreciate what you've done to prevent errors, but I need more."

Resist this temptation. Drop any use of the word "but" in your message. Give your rewarding words a chance to be internalized, so they become part of the person's own long term self motivation for safe behavior.

Don't misplace the focus

If a material reward accompanies social approval, words of appreciation can become less significant. This, in turn, lessens the impact on one's self-reinforcement system. Tangibles can add to the quality of interpersonal recognition if they are delivered as tokens of appreciation. But they must not be viewed as a payoff for the safety-related behavior — only as a symbol of what was accomplished to reduce risk and improve patient care.

Spread the word

Sometimes people are suspicious of praise when it's delivered face-to-face. Is there an ulterior motive, another agenda at work? Perhaps some favor is expected in return. Or maybe the recognition is seen merely as an extension of a communication exercise.

Suppose someone other than a safety coach or patient-safety leader spreads the word through a unit about the superb job a coworker did spotting a potential medication error and speaking up. People will likely consider this kind of "grassroots" recognition genuine. This pass-along recognition can also build a sense of belonging or group cohesion among individuals. Gossip can be beneficial — if it is positive. We call it "positive gossip."

7 Ten coaching guidelines
Time-tested and state-of-the-art

These ten guidelines for implementing an effective safety coaching process to prevent risks and protect patients were developed and refined from studying the trials and tribulations of more than 100 industrial clients of the leading-edge consulting firm Safety Performance Solutions (SPS). We're convinced they reflect the state-of-the-art in safety coaching.

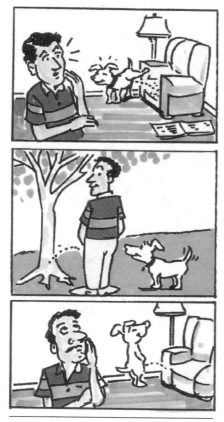

Training without education can be ineffective.

1) *Teach principles*

There is a difference between education and training. Education explains "why" and training shows "how." Motivation to learn what to do — the procedures — can come from understanding the underlying rationale — the principles. Before people are trained on our ACTS (Acting-Coaching-Thinking-Seeing) process, for example, they should be educated on the philosophical foundations of People-Based Patient Safety™. That's why you are reading this book.

When participants learn and accept the principles behind any type of safety initiative, they can help define and refine tools and techniques applicable for their units. Such involvement in designing process steps facilitates empowerment and ownership — the next guideline.

2) *Empower employees*

"Empowerment" has become a cheap cliché in cultures where it gets only lip service. Just remember, genuine empowerment is not something that can be handed over to employees. People feel enabled to act to improve patient safety when they feel a personal sense of ownership for the issue. We're not talking about management abdicating its responsibilities and adding to employees' "to do" lists. And we're not talking about responsibilities in the sense of complying with accreditation rules.

Once people are given the green light to design, implement, evaluate, and refine a patient-safety process, they acquire a special degree of ownership. It can be a fragile feeling in the beginning, something that needs to be nurtured by both coaches and organization leaders.

3) Give 'em a choice

Choice, involvement and ownership: each supports the other two. More of one influences more of the others.

Choice is energizing. Research has shown that even insignificant choice benefits commitment and human performance. For example, Safety Action Teams at the Children's Hospitals and Clinics of Minnesota begin to take control of their work environment by reviewing incidents — or what the hospital calls "learning reports" — and choosing one local, high-risk safety issue to address over the course of a year. Solutions developed by the various teams are judged and recognized in an annual competition.

But keep this in mind: too much choice, too much of a good thing, can actually be detrimental. In studying the successes and failures of SPS clients, we found that safety coaching programs labeled "completely voluntary" were generally not as successful as programs introduced with the explicit expectation that everyone will get involved to some degree. That's the way it works at Sentara Healthcare, where behavior-based expectations for error prevention are intended for use by all 12,000 employees.

Provide structure and direction, but accompany your advice with opportunities to select among alternative action plans. Maintain appropriate balance between organizational structure and individual choice.

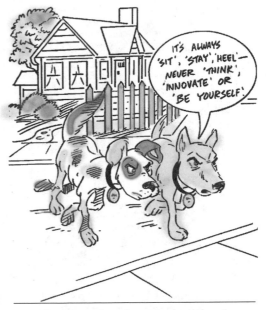

Command and control without choice stifle creativity.

That's what the Children's Hospitals and Clinics of Minnesota does. Those local or micro safety priorities chosen by the Safety Action Teams are balanced with system-wide macro targets that all teams work on, such as patient and information transfers between departments.

4) Facilitate supportive managers

A "hands off" policy does not work. Let's face reality: People give priority to the aspects of their jobs that get attention from on high. People do what they believe they need to do in order to please the powers that be. "I know what I should do is model all the time," acknowledges one hospital CEO we interviewed. "A significant part of what any CEO does is symbolic. People look at the CEO and make interpretations all the time," he told us.

Yes, self-directed, personally responsible behavior is best. But often behavior must start as other-directed. (Recall the different types of behavior from Chapter 2 on Acting.) Before people can appreciate the natural supportive consequences of a People-Based Patient Safety™ process, they usually need to be held accountable for carrying out certain expectations.

5) Go easy on punishment

We discussed the disadvantages of traditional discipline in the previous chapter on Acting. It's worth repeating: If you connect blame, punishment, or any negative consequence to any aspect of your employee-driven and management-supported patient-safety activity, you can kill the entire process. Punishment hammers feelings of trust and tears down a commitment to risk reduction.

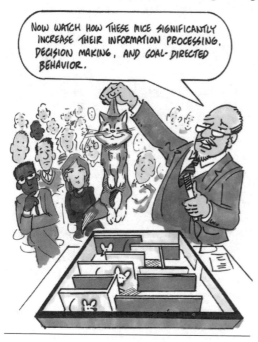

NOW WATCH HOW THESE MICE SIGNIFICANTLY INCREASE THEIR INFORMATION PROCESSING, DECISION MAKING, AND GOAL-DIRECTED BEHAVIOR.

Punishment is efficient but has negative side effects.

If you want to use negative consequences to motivate compliance, do so at your own risk. But be sure to administer discipline policy independently of all People-Based Patient Safety™ activities.

We prefer this approach: Finding low incident reporting rates or at-risk behavior is not cause for breaking out the rod — it pinpoints opportunities for improvement. What suppresses reporting? Why are hand-offs haphazard? Open and frank conversation about areas of concern is much more likely than punishment to increase mindful commitment to change, and to activate peer support for specific improvement targets.

6) Stick to the facts

At first, coaching often feels awkward. So from the start it's critical to realize the safety coach, unlike the typical athletic coach, is not responsible for correcting behavior. Take the pressure off your coaches. Unless it's a case where harm to a patient is imminent (and direct intervention is absolutely required), coaching relies on the informal give-and-take of interpersonal conversation. The focus is on questioning, listening, and flushing out information about system pressures and problems, as well as human dynamics that cause risks to patient and staff safety. We're talking about such risks as taking shortcuts, ignoring protocols, and devising ad hoc schemes that circumvent the system.

In these discussions, no direct disapproval of any at-risk behavior is offered — again, unless imminent harm to a patient is clear. Coaching is not about debating or arguing. This is nondirective persuasion and guidance. There is no peer pressure. Only self-accountability matters here. Any lasting change in behavior is self-directed, facilitated by a coach's observations and suggestions.

7) *Place trust above accuracy*

As a coach at a VA hospital in the Pittsburgh area, Peter Perreiah announces to the staff in advance that observation sessions will be conducted in an effort to shape the behaviors needed to lower the rate of hospital-acquired infections. Since this could easily lead to "showcase" behaviors, why announce observations in advance?

Coaches who sleuth around and complete observations on the sly are conducting nothing less than a "gotcha" program. Ambushing employees is a surefire way to undermine trust, involvement, and ownership. A "gotcha" program" might give you lower, more accurate "percent safe" scores of target behaviors, but at the expense of the cooperation needed to prevent medical errors and protect patients.

An observation process holds people accountable to perform tasks as safely as they know how. Even when they know they are being observed, employees will still take certain risks. When they learn ways to be safer under open, transparent circumstances, workers truly add new behavioral patterns to their knowledge base.

8) *Avoid paralysis by analysis*

Most records of behavioral observations are likely to be biased and unreliable. They are typically obtained under unnatural conditions. As mentioned, observations are often announced beforehand, and there is a tendency by coaches or observers to overlook at-risk behavior, especially when feedback is to immediately follow.

In industry, most companies chart the number of safe and at-risk behaviors observed to measure changes in behavior patterns over time, and to compare teams and departments. But don't get hung up on chasing numbers. The coaching process, with its conversational give and take, is more powerful than tallying up observations.

One-to-one coaching demonstrates peer support, develops interpersonal trust, and helps to cultivate the kind of learning-oriented organization that brings out the best in people. The process teaches staff they can be "unconsciously incompetent" and they need feedback from others to improve. This leads to interdependency — people contributing diverse talents and relying on each other to make the whole organization greater than the sum of its parts.

9) *Refine your process*

With experience, behavioral coaches become more adept at noticing subtle features of safe versus at-risk work practices. For instance, some of Sentara Healthcare's Behavior-Based Expectations look for evidence of questioning attitudes, verifying and validating, and clearing your head before taking on a critical job.

Continue to assess the behavioral and attitudinal impact of your coaching procedures. Evaluating people's opinions and attitudes about a behavioral coaching process requires conversations with both participants and nonparticipants. These should occur in group and individual one-to-one sessions.

10) Focus on people factors

There's more to coaching than observing. People-Based Patient Safety™ coaching applies empathy, facilitation, advocacy, optimism, and negotiation to change not only how people act, think and recognize risks on their own, but how they interact and work together as a team to achieve patient-safety goals.

8 How to get the most from your teams
From "radical individualism" to interdependence

We hear all the talk about the need for collaboration and interdependence in healthcare, just like you do. We see the proliferation of patient-safety audit teams, rapid response teams, performance improvement teams, root-cause analysis teams, too. But as anyone who's ever tried to coach a team knows, be it a young girls' soccer team, a church fundraising team, or a safety team, it's not easy to get teams working the way you want them to.

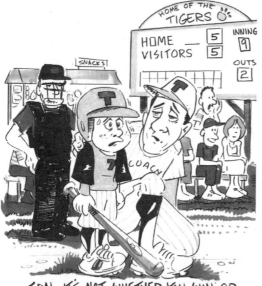

SON, IT'S NOT WHETHER YOU WIN OR LOSE... UNLESS YOU WANT DADDY'S LOVE.

A win/lose mindset conflicts with interdependency.

Teamwork just doesn't come naturally to most of us. After all, look at how we've been raised. "Be independent," we're told from early on. We compete with other individuals to get ahead, whether at work or at play. "Nice guys finish last." A win-lose, me-first mindset is promoted by everything from the grades we get in school to salary promotions at work.

It's surely promoted in medicine. "The culture of medicine is one of radical individualism," says risk communication expert Peter Sandman. "Every doc is a rugged individualist, and patients like the ideal of their doc being decisive, self-confident, their own person."

Learning to work effectively as a team takes patience and practice, just like with sports squads. Teamwork calls for compromises and sacrifices that most of us are not accustomed to making. Sometimes bureaucratic red tape, policies or procedures, can tangle up teams and slow down their progress. But those obstacles can be easier to remove than smoothing out the individual differences that can inhibit teamwork.

Integrating a group of people into a team requires attention to each person's perspective of what's going on, their expectations for the team and their special roles, how they communicate, their relations with other team members, and how their behavior — bullying or diffident, for example — affects team interplay.

We're talking about recognizing and changing the perspectives each person brings to a team — those powerful personal biases, beliefs and values. Whatever your attitude is toward a particular experience, or your expectation of how things will work out, that's your perspective:

"Sorry. Not now. I don't have time to be part of your team."

"Sorry, but my schedule's just too packed to take on any more meetings. Plus, I'm in and out of the hospital and I'm never sure when I'll be there."

Personal perceptions influence the way we view a situation, and what we extract from it. As a result, we often experience what we expect to happen, and learn what we expect to learn. It's a self-fulfilling prophecy. We act a certain way to be consistent with our world view, and so increase the odds that what we believe will actually occur.

And let's face it, many of us don't have a strong belief in the efficacy of teams. Too much squabbling. Too many egos. Too much wasted time.

So if you plan to use teams to tackle patient-safety issues, one of your first tasks is to figure out how to shift those perspectives everyone brings to the table. In healthcare, most people bring expectations of and beliefs in authority and autonomy to the table. That's what has led over time to systems that are often a loose collection of fiefdoms almost "independently owned and operated" by units and departments. "Silos" the quality experts call them.

How do you get people out of silos and into teams? You go to work on perceptions and expectations. To put it in behavioral terms, set goals based on actions, then watch how achieving those goals leads to new ways of thinking. In other words, when people get involved in a process that requires interdependency and they see the benefits of this process, they will change their perspectives. They will have acted their way into a new line of thinking.

Promoting high-reliability surgery: An operating room pilot project aimed at promoting teamwork at the Kaiser Permanente Anaheim (California) Medical Center used a behavioral checklist and goal setting to reduce errors and improve safety attitudes. A team including surgeons, anesthetists, operating-room nurses, technicians, and managers used a one-page checklist to guide preparations for cases.

Similar to a preflight checklist in aviation, each form was adapted to the needs of each case, indicating the roles of team members in each case. The checklist was posted throughout the operating theatre as a mental prompt.

After a six-month trial of pre-operative safety briefings — "time outs" — using the checklists, improved performance relating to four outcome measures (or goals) was achieved. Wrong-site surgeries, which occurred three times in the prior year, were eliminated. Reports of close calls increased, suggesting greater situational awareness. Sixty-three percent of team members rated the operating room safety climate as good, compared to 51 percent before the pilot. And nursing staff turnover, an indicator of staff morale, decreased from 23 percent before the intervention to 7 percent.[6]

Case study *Safety Action Teams at the Children's Hospitals and Clinics of Minnesota*

Julianne M. Morath, M.S., R.N., is the chief operating officer for Children's Hospitals and Clinics of Minnesota and co-author of the book, *To Do No Harm*, published in 2005.

Q *How did you develop your Safety Action Teams?*

A *Initially our patient-safety plan was led by executives. We examined the model of the distance between the blunt (management) and sharp (front-line) ends of our system, and how to close the distance through an architecture of engagement. One nurse piloted our first Safety Action Team (SAT) in the hematology/oncology unit. This was in 2000. We now have 28 teams, in both clinical and support areas such as environmental sciences and materials management. All of them are voluntarily, and all are multi-disciplinary.*

Teams typically have 5–10 members, and can include a physician, a pharmacist, several nurses, the health unit coordinator or secretary, and a respiratory therapist. It depends on the unit. The team convenes a minimum of once a month in usually 60–90 minute meetings to work on patient-safety issues local to them. These targets can be identified through the reporting system, which we call "Patient Safety Learning Reports," and by reviewing entries on our "Good Catch" logs, where staff informally jot down patient-safety issues and ideas.

Teams work on one self-selected, locally relevant issue per year. For example, the hematology/oncology program decided its process for administering chemotherapy needed to be improved. The process caused delays for children and families, resulting in chemotherapy initiated late in the evening. The team changed the entire admissions process to provide care while expert resources were available on site; overtime was eliminated; and the new process enhanced family satisfaction.

We have also chartered all SATs to tackle a system-wide issue, such as reducing risks during transfer of care. In this case, teams worked together, because you have transfers from the emergency department to the inpatient environment, from the operating room to recovery and postoperative care. We also looked at rounds and sign outs — information hand-offs between providers. We have seen improvements. For instance, mislabeled specimens have been reduced by greater than 80 percent in a year.

Teams are fueled by the use of rapid cycle improvement methods. They receive continuous feedback on their progress toward fixing a problem. (Rapid cycles are driven by three questions: What are we trying to accomplish? What changes can we make that will result in improvement? How will we know a change is an improvement? These questions lead to a cycle of plan, do, study and act.)

Teams are also fueled by healthy competition. We have a juried competition each year — a poster session at our annual safety conference. Each team displays a poster describing its work in the past year. We recognize a first-place winner and two finalists. Entries are judged on 1) identifying a problem informed by data, 2) use of rapid cycle improvement, 3) rigorous analysis of outcome, 4) improvement in outcome, and 5) replicability.

We fund the winning team to go to a national patient-safety conference, such as the National Patient Safety Foundation annual congress. Finalists receive a monetary award in the range of $200–$500 per team.

If a team is stalling out or unable to initiate a project, we'll help out. If there's no progress toward a goal, or the team can't agree on the scope of its activity, we'll have an executive resource, patient-safety specialist, or performance improvement specialist work with the team to design their project and implement it.

You usually find informal leaders step forward to direct a team. Sometimes they might be encouraged to take the lead by a manager. The leaders of the SATs convene quarterly as part of our architecture of learning. They share what they've learned and spread innovations and best practices.

Shifting perspectives

Consider this principle of human nature while reviewing five changes in thinking, or perspective, needed for high-performance teamwork. We can literally act ourselves into becoming a better team player — if we follow these interconnected transitions.

1 — From individual to team performance. Traditional work holds people accountable for their own behavior. Effective teamwork, though, requires mutual accountability. It's not "What you do is what you get," but rather "How you collaborate with others is what the group gets." Effective collaboration nets greater performance results than what individuals can do by themselves. This is a synergistic outcome.

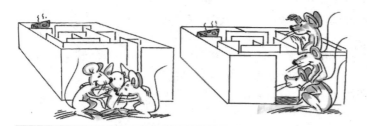

Trust, cooperation and interdependency reap synergistic rewards.

2 — From individual jobs to team tasks. This synergy occurs when each team member contributes individual talent and effort to improve team performance. Team members receive task assignments from each other, and carry out their responsibilities to support the rest of the team. Teamwork requires a shift from working exclusively to achieve personal goals to working to achieve shared team goals. This takes a belief in the power of teamwork, a commitment toward the team's mission, and trust that every team member will do his or her part to meet team objectives.

3 — From competitive rewards to rewards for cooperation. It takes a special mindset to revel in the accomplishments of a team effort, especially in medicine with its reliance on practice specialties. When team members value their mutual purpose and believe teammates will cooperate to achieve shared goals, they put forth their best efforts. And when they see cooperation pay off, they develop a unique appreciation for teamwork. They feel personally recognized when their team is rewarded. Then they cooperate more to fulfill their team's next objectives.

4 — From self-dependence to team-dependence. We come into this world dependent on others to take care of us. As children we depend on our family for all our basic life needs. As adolescents, however, we look for opportunities to be on our own. The primary mission in life for most teenagers, it seems, is to resist dependency and assert independence. This reliance on self rather than others is promoted and reinforced throughout our culture. It's certainly fueled in the highly competitive, individualistic culture of medicine.

"I've spent six years trying to engage physicians in patient-safety work," says the chief operating officer of a 300-bed hospital. "It takes renewed effort every day."

One reason for that is high-performance teamwork requires a dependency perspective. Of course in healthcare, professionals have supreme confidence in their own problem-solving skills, and many question the ability of, or need for, others to help. The notion of dependency is alien and unappealing.

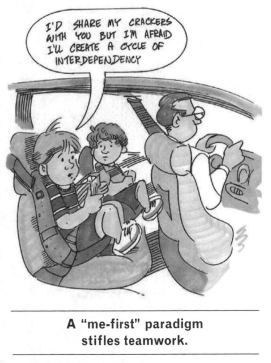

**A "me-first" paradigm
stifles teamwork.**

Well, it might seem like regression, but it's really progression. In fact, it's more appropriate to consider teamwork a shift to interdependence rather than dependence. That's because the dependency between team members is reciprocal. While you depend on team members to complete their task assignments, others depend on you to do your part. We're moving from independence to interdependency here. The more you trust the ability and intentions of the other individuals on your team, the more you depend on your teammates for their contributions — and the more you feel obligated to complete your own task assignments.

Let's face facts: the myriad patient-safety issues challenging healthcare systems will never be solved using the old individualistic model of medicine. Medical errors rarely result from the actions of one person, and reducing errors requires contributions from a multi-disciplinary team of caregivers. "Caregivers know where the failures are, where the potential to harm exists," says Rosemary Gibson, author of *Wall of Silence*. "They know they could do a better job, and they know they need help."

5 — From one-to-one communication to group interaction. You tap into those feelings and build trust and interdependency through interpersonal communication. Some of this certainly happens through one-to-one interaction. But the synergistic power of teamwork is more readily realized through effective team discussions. Through group interaction, individuals come to see how their diverse talents combine to solve problems and achieve positive outcomes. It takes time to cultivate group cohesion and feelings of belonging. Many times coaches or facilitators will jump in to steer the team through its early stages of forming and storming.[7]

Another value of group interaction is that it can present individuals with a global overview of the synergies inherent in healthcare systems. From pre-op care, to surgery and post-op care, synergistic teamwork occurs everywhere. It's possible an individual healthcare professional does not see this interdependency. It's easy to miss the forest from the trees.

"The individual physician might believe his own personal concern for patient safety is sufficient," says a physician in a group practice on the west coast. "For any one physician working in his or her little sphere, medical errors may seem infrequent. But if you work in an oversight capacity in a hospital and review all the mistakes and errors that occur, you get a different consciousness."

Participation in teams can elevate that consciousness, too.

Case study CUSPs at The Johns Hopkins Hospital

Lori Ann Paine, M.S., R.N., is the patient-safety coordinator for The Johns Hopkins Hospital.

Q *Describe your Comprehensive Unit-Based Safety Programs, or CUSPs.*

A *"Culture lives locally" is the mantra of Bryan Sexton, who works with us here as assistant professor in the Department of Anesthesiology and Critical Care Medicine. He is researching patient-safety climate and teamwork climates in intensive care units.*

CUSPs are a model for creating a positive safety culture at the unit level. It involves assessing the unit culture of safety, educating staff, finding and fixing defects, and building teamwork in partnership with senior leaders. They are now in place in at least 20 units at The Johns Hopkins Hospital.

To begin with, I lead one-hour "Safety Science 101" sessions for unit staff. Frontline people think sometimes they already "get" safety — they know where the fire exits and extinguishers are. But they don't understand the importance of communication and teamwork in ensuring safety.

As part of our initial unit surveying, we ask, "Where is the next patient in this unit going to be harmed? What can we do to prevent that harm?"

The answers they give are fairly predictable: medication error, falls and infection. Almost always some form of communication breakdown comes up, between nurses and physicians or residents and physicians. It's better to allow frontline people to express their concerns than to have "suits" — executives — come in with all the answers, saying, "Well, isn't it obvious?"

*We partner a senior executive with each CUSP to make rounds, iden-
tify problems, and work on an agenda to make improvements. There is a
direct dose-response relationship at work here: the more frequent a CUSP
team works with a senior executive, the higher the scores are from that unit
on the Safety Attitude Questionnaire.*

*Executives help find early wins with patient safety, things that can be
pounded out today — the low-hanging fruit. They can also cut through turf
battles and red tape to get what's needed, something like a computer perhaps.*

*We challenge each CUSP to find and fix a defect a month. Problems are
identified through our reporting system, our staff safety surveys, a complaint
from a patient, or a sentinel event. This system of challenges gives structure
to each unit's patient-safety work, and keeps safety momentum moving forward. It can be something as simple as speeding up the time it takes
medications to get to the unit from the pharmacy. Then we rigorously assess
data, pre- and post-intervention.*

*Much of what we learn or do in one unit is transferable to other units.
Sometimes units will say they're different, it couldn't possibly work with
them. But we're all one large system, and the problems can seem overwhelming. CUSPs are a way of improving the culture of safety from the
bottom up, one unit at a time.*

9 Responding to resistance
Don't lecture, don't pry... take a deep breath

Of course anyone who conducts a meeting or shepherds a team along is going
to be on the receiving end of some cynical and disturbing statements. Safety
coaches, meeting facilitators and team leaders must know how to react. Let's
discuss guidelines for constructive reaction when these situations flare up.

Typical reactions

When someone complains with such emotional outbursts as, "I'm quitting
the team," "It's out of our hands," or "It will never work here," the adult counselor in us comes out. We're ready to jump in with quick-fix advice. But hold
on. This advice comes from a selective interpretation of what we hear, filtered
through our personal views. Regardless, we proceed to lecture, like an adult to
a child. We tell the person what he or she should or should not do. To make
matters worse, we often preface our unsolicited counseling with phrases like "If
I were you," or "When I was in a similar situation, I..."

If we don't lecture, we might pry — another typical reaction to signals of distress. We take a radical statement like "I'm going to quit the team" at face value and follow it by asking, "Why?" We're trying to quickly get to the bottom or root cause of the person's problem. We think we'll be able to solve their distress if we know more about it. So we interrogate the individual, true detective style, with specific questions in order to evaluate the situation and provide advice.

We have a lot of practice with this style of grilling, so much that it becomes a natural communication pattern. Think about your interactions with family members at home. Sometimes we know a family member, such as a young child, well enough to probe, evaluate, and counsel. But this approach often misses the mark, even at home. Your premature guidance is frequently off-base and resisted. A verbal investigation implies blame or judgment, and often mutes the other person.

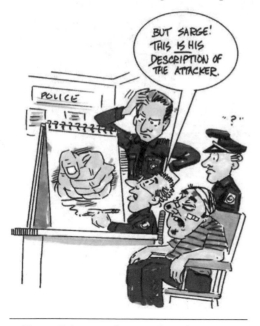

At the root of our reaction is "autobiographical bias." You see, we try to evaluate and guide others using our own experiences as a map. We use "selective perception" to put what someone says into our personal frame of reference. We respond to what's relevant to us, and base advice on our past experiences and biases.

This kind of reaction to another person's "issues" is likely to be off-target. Even if well-intentioned advice is appropriate, it's not likely to be accepted because it probably comes across as biased. It might even be perceived as cold, uncaring.

Empathic coaches understand the other person's perspective.

So slow down. If we want people in a meeting or on a team to listen to our advice and accept guidance, we have to resist the quick-fix response to problems when they crop up.

It takes time to understand a problem or assess a situation from another person's perspective instead of our own. This calls for active listening. We need to grasp the other person's biased viewpoint before making interpretations and suggestions. We need to keep our own ego in check, allowing the other person to share their true perceptions and feelings. Premature probing, evaluating, and advising — a rush to judge — will probably cut the person off from revealing private thoughts and emotions.

It's possible, even likely, initial statements from a troubled coworker do not reflect the real issue. To say, "I'm quitting the team," is a broad, blunt statement, and might even be an over-reaction to get your attention. Much more information is needed for you to possibly understand what's going on behind that kind of declaration and offer useful and acceptable advice.

Keep in mind, people are usually reluctant to reveal their deeper emotions — even to family members — even though we can't really help unless there is such self-disclosure. To show you truly care, you need to be an engaged, empathetic listener.

Dale Carnegie wrote about the value of active listening more than 50 years ago in his classic book, *How to Win Friends and Influence People*.[8] His wisdom is reflected in the writing of many contemporary authors, including Stephen Covey's fifth habit of highly effective people, "Seek First to Understand... Then to be Understood."[9] Carnegie, Covey, and others offer the same basic strategies for active listening; if you've had any training in effective communication, you've received the same advice.

Listening guidelines

Let's review these guidelines for reacting to resistance with four easy-to-remember words, each beginning with the letter "R." In today's healthcare world (or just about any work environment) rife with frustration, anxiety and stress, we need to be teachers and users of active listening principles.

1 — Repeat

This is the same technique used to verify medications. Simply mimic or repeat what you hear using the same basic words as the speaker. This clarifies you heard correctly, and most importantly, prompts the person to say more. Remember, the purpose of active listening is to persuade the other person to say more so you can get at the root of the problem.

So if a team member tells you he is quitting, you might repeat, "You're quitting?" This shows you're attentive and interested, and waiting for more information. Hearing how drastic the declaration sounds, the person might reply, "Well, at least I feel like quitting." Then what would you say? Following this repeat technique, you would say, "You mean you feel like quitting?" Or, you might use different words to echo the same meaning. This is the next active listening technique.

2 — Rephrase

Instead of mimicking what you hear, you might rephrase the words. In our example, you might say, "You mean you don't like working on this team anymore?" By putting the statement in your own words, you show genuine interest while also asking for more information. You're also checking for understanding. If you can rephrase the statement correctly, you have accurately received and interpreted what's been said.

Suppose he clarifies, "Well, it's not that I don't like working on the team, it's just that our lack of progress gets me so frustrated at times, I feel like quitting." Now your coworker has revealed a more specific aspect of the problem. What do you say next?

You could use the repeat strategy and return with, "Our lack of progress gets you down?" Or you could attempt to rephrase with something like, "You mean our slow progress makes you so impatient it saps your motivation?" Perhaps this statement calls for the next "R" of active listening — ratification.

3 — *Ratify*

Here you offer words that show empathy for what is being said, and this in turn, encourages more explanation. In our example, you might ratify your appreciation of the statement by saying, "I know the feeling, I've been frustrated with progress myself at times and wonder whether my efforts to promote more teamwork are worth it."

At this point, you might be tempted to jump in with probing questions to find out more about what your team member sees as a lack of team progress. What kind of expectations did this individual have that caused the emotional upheaval? What makes this person different, leading to a decision to quit while other team members are hanging in?

Resist the temptation to overreach. More active listening could reveal problems beyond the issue of "progress." Perhaps it's not the amount of progress per se, but a particular team assignment. Or the problem might stem from interactions with another team member, or personal issues away from the team, or from feelings of inadequate contributions, including a perceived loss of confidence, self-esteem, or personal control.

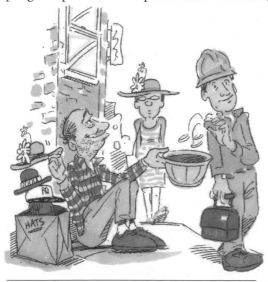

Empathy can be rewarding.

The bottom line is that a person's distress signals can emanate from many sources, and these will not surface quickly in one-to-one conversation. Even if the relevant causes of a problem are truthfully disclosed, it's unlikely you could give immediate advice that is both useful and acted upon. Usually, the best we can do is listen actively with repeat, rephrase, and ratify strategies in order to get the problem out in the open.

Ultimately, we want people to express the full range of their true feelings.

4 — Reflect

When people reflect on their inner feelings about a situation, they are at the personal root of the problem. Such self-disclosure can lead to insight into the true cause of the problem, for both speaker and listener, and suggest strategies for intervention. However, even with outer layers of the onion peeled away, it's usually better to let the speaker consider various solutions.

If you've been an actively-caring listener, you might eventually get the ultimate reward for your sensitivity, patience, and emotional intelligence. The speaker will ask you for specific advice.

When you hear words like, "What do you think I should do?" you have mastered active listening. You have shown you actively care, and now your direction will likely be most relevant, understood, and accepted. Actually, a better description for this highest level of listening is "empathic listening."

10   The value of story-telling

Nothing connects to the true purpose of patient safety like a story

"A lot of coaching is telling stories and analyzing them. It's not about counting things." — Martin J. Hatlie, president, Partnership for Patient Safety

Want to pull people out of their silos? Open eyes? Keep people in their seats at meetings? Want to coalesce a team around patient safety? Use the ancient art of story-telling. And infuse your story with passion and genuine concern.

As Hatlie explains, most medical "failures" lend themselves to open-ended narrative treatments, involving as they do a series of events not easily captured on forms. They require the kind of context provided by story-telling.

And stories of errors and near-errors strike a realistic chord with caregivers. Personal stories draw people in, especially when they can relate and put themselves in the plot line. "You've got to appeal to where people live," says Rosemary Gibson. "Everyone wants to feel good about saving lives. Make your appeals relevant to their work and their patients." Nothing can connect to that sense of purpose and dedication more than a story such as this one:

"Every parent's nightmare"

This edited story comes from a posting on the PULSE patient-safety organization web site, written by a young father following the loss of his 13-month-old daughter.

"When our 13-month-old daughter was brought into the emergency room we were told the shunt, placed in her head at birth, was in failure, her condition was 'emergent,' and she required immediate surgery. We were then told that since the OR was too busy and due to the late hour and it being the weekend, she was being bumped that evening and would have to wait until the next morning for surgery.

"To compound the problem, she was not even placed in an intensive care unit, nor was she properly monitored while she awaited surgery.

"Prior to being placed in her room, the resident neurosurgeon working that evening at the hospital paged the attending neurosurgeon who was supposed to do the surgery and was on call. He had previously given an order to the resident to tap the shunt, which the resident did, but the shunt was dry and no fluid was obtained. He repeatedly paged the attending neurosurgeon, but he had put his pager on vibrate as he went into a supermarket, and then went home and fell asleep.

"The resident neurosurgeon also ordered blood tests, which were taken that evening. They showed my daughter had critical carbon dioxide levels, as well as abnormal potassium and sodium levels. Nobody, including the resident neurosurgeon, bothered to inquire about, acknowledge or address these abnormal results.

"No doctor ever examined my daughter from the time she was admitted to the time she went into respiratory arrest — 12:20 a.m. to 6:20 a.m.

"I lived every parent's nightmare of losing a child and this is especially difficult because our child should be alive today. Because of medical errors, she is not. This is why I'm fighting for patients' rights and ways to prevent this senseless tragedy from happening to another child or family."

"The board was blown away"

Jeff Cooper, Ph.D., director of biomedical engineering for Partners HealthCare System in Boston, once took a group of board members on a retreat where they heard several hours of stories from patients and the families of patients. "These were powerful stories," he recalls. "Two were overt errors. In one case a husband died. In another, a son was left paralyzed. The board was blown away. The response was far more than I anticipated."

Of course, case reports have long been the focus of morbidity and mortality conferences. Today detailed analyses of errors leading to patient harm, or near harm, can be found all over the internet on patient-safety web sites. An excellent resource is the Agency for Healthcare Research & Quality's *Morbidity and Mortality Rounds* on the Web.

But the more personal and relevant your patient-safety stories — like those heard on Dr. Cooper's retreat — the more you'll pull people in. And you don't have to be the story-teller. If you can arrange it, have patients themselves, or their families, recount encounters with medical error. Or have staff talk about their personal experiences.

In healthcare, everyone has been touched by error and likely has a story to tell. Atul Gawande in his book, *Complications*, concedes, "The fact is virtually everyone who cares for hospital patients will make serious mistakes, and even commit acts of negligence, every year."[10]

But how do you get people to open up and share, when many are quite naturally anxious about looking dumb or careless? Perhaps they fear retaliation or reprimand, or possible malpractice legal action.

Here's a thought: If you want to arrange for public disclosures at your patient-safety meetings, put the spotlight on close calls. We all have close calls or "near misses" of some sort on a regular basis, and in each case we can imagine a worst-case scenario if it were not for luck or timing.

There is no threat of malpractice legal action if the story is a close call — if harm never reached the patient. And discussing close calls and ways to prevent them is the best way to avoid the worst-case scenario. Plus, this optimal scare tactic works when those involved are asked to identify ways to prevent the error or tragedy.

For this kind of story-telling to be effective, it's important the staff listening to the account of near-harm believe the prevention solutions offered in the follow-up discussion will actually work. This is a true definition of feeling empowered. It requires a person to answer "yes" to three questions: *Can I do it?* (self-efficacy); *Will it work?* (response efficacy); and *Is it worth it?* (outcome expectancy). The third question is the most challenging, because it is the motivation factor.

Bottom line: use personal stories of close calls to activate personal emotions and caring, and perhaps fear. Then provide an intervention that can prevent future occurrences of the close call or error. Teach the intervention technique so people can do it and believe it will work.

11 Is your audience ready for your story?

Your ability to persuade depends on "fit"

Personal testimonies are one form of story-telling. But you can also craft stories that carry a broader message or theme for patient safety.

Here's what we're getting at. As a coach for safety, or as a patient-safety coordinator or director, you are in the position of being what Howard Gardner in his book *Leading Minds*[11] calls an "indirect leader." You influence the thinking and behavior of your organization and its people through the indirect application of your patient-safety expertise and insights.

Direct leaders, in contrast, typically lack astute knowledge of any given subject area. But they have their hands on the levers of power, such as CEOs and heads of state.

Central to Gardner's thesis is that leaders, whether their style is direct or indirect, must have a story to relate, and an audience ready to hear it, if they are to succeed.

By "story," Gardner means a central theme or message. But, as he says, it is no mere headline or slogan. It's a perspective — a conviction — communicated not just in words, but actions.

A leader's ability to persuade and be effective depends on fit, writes Gardner. The same goes for your prevention of errors to improve patient safety. The story needs to make sense to audience members, in terms of where they have been and where they want to go.

Think of FDR's "We have nothing to fear…" speech at the outset of World War II, JFK's "Ask not what your country can do for you" message at the dawn of the idealistic 1960s, and George W. Bush's reassurances after 9/11.

Think of your own patient-safety "story" and the audience you're trying to reach. How good is the fit? Are they ready to hear your message? After all, many safety stories — in and out of healthcare — promote the themes of obligation, commitment and responsibility.

You need to be aware of several barriers to safety-related story-telling:

• *First, consider your audience.* Or rather, your audiences — administrators, physicians, nurses, various specialists, and various employees who service the hospital, from food service to equipment maintenance. Are these people poised to respond to repeated presentations of your core patient-safety message?

For as Gardner writes, "Even the most eloquent story is stillborn in the absence of an audience ready to hear it."

We could have a problem here. Actually, several problems relating to the promotion of patient safety.

For one, the personal experiences of your audience members may not align with the safety message. Medical failures usually happen to someone else. Over time statistics show that most frontline caregivers will be touched by error[12], but it is not a day-to-day, top-of-mind thought.

• *Timing is everything.* Safety stories resonate most powerfully when the audience is living the story — NASA after the *Columbia* disaster, or a hospital after a highly publicized and preventable patient death. Then the fit, the readiness to listen and respond, is acute.

But long-term chances of success are greater if your story can take root in a non-crisis situation, through sustained, concentrated effort. Sentinel events and fatalities, unfortunately, lend themselves to emotional knee-jerk reactions, often resulting in temporary improvement, which is neither significant nor enduring.

• *Another challenge: competition from other stories.* Consider some of the stories competing for the attention and commitment of your managers and employees (adapted from a list compiled by risk communication expert Peter Sandman):

"We've got deadlines, budgets, real problems," says a COO.

"We've got good patient-safety grades already," says a department head.

"If they just paid attention, no one would get hurt," says a shift supervisor.

"Management doesn't care about patient safety," says an employee.

• *Finally, beware of disengagement.* Consider a poll by the Society of Human Resource Management and CNN.[13] When asked to rank 21 aspects of their daily work life in terms of importance to personal job satisfaction, a random nationwide sample of more than 600 employees put relationships with coworkers 20th, job-specific training 19th, and contribution of work to the organization's business goals 17th.

Ouch.

OK, now the good news. Here is how you can strengthen your patient-safety story for its broadest possible impact:

• *Build your expertise and credibility.* A story is unlikely to achieve any credibility or gain traction unless the author's track record is one of high quality.[14] Here, patient-safety mavens with experience on the frontlines and access to networks, resources and knowledge unavailable to the rest of the organization have an advantage.

• *Authenticity.* Patient-safety leaders are the real deal. Their passion and determination propel them to live out and project their stories — their vision and themes and even specific actions and attitudes they require — every day. So they wear gloves, gowns and masks when needed, follow all safety-related procedures, pursue patient-safety audit findings until closure, etc. In some cases, their story can even be strengthened if they own up to unsafe thinking and actions of the past — a "counter-story."[15]

In contrast, if the leader seems to contradict his story by his overt behavior, if he appears hypocritical, the story won't be convincing over the long run.

• *Natural tendencies.* See if you can relate to some of the qualities of an "exemplary leader": Possessing a keen interest in, and understanding of, other people; general energy and resourcefulness; conviction that one's own insights are well motivated and likely to be effective; and concerned with moral issues.[16]

Indeed, these are all common markers of effective patient-safety leaders.

• *Inclusiveness.* The most influential stories encourage individuals to think of themselves as part of a broader community.[17] Think of the appeals of FDR, JFK, Reagan, Martin Luther King, and Gandhi. Think of all that's been said in patient-safety literature about belongingness, ownership, teamwork and building a safety culture. Safety's message is naturally inclusive. It applies to all of us, everywhere, all the time.

Take a look at your safety story-telling. What are your themes and methods of delivering your messages? Study your audiences, and the counter-stories in your workplace that compete for attention. Leverage those factors — credibility, timing, authenticity — that work in your favor for changing attitudes and behaviors related to reducing errors and improving patient care.

12 How to coach patients
How to fuel their active involvement

Many coaching and communications skills we've discussed here certainly can be leveraged in the current campaign to get patients more involved in their own care and personal safety. Patients are being prepped to[18]:
  • Speak up if you have questions or concerns. (JCAHO Speak Up)
  • Be an active member of your healthcare team. (AHRQ 20 Tips)
  • Encourage care providers to adopt safety-promoting practices, such as hand-washing, or confirming patient identification.
  • Report anything unusual to your doctor, such as any changes in your condition. (NPSF Your Role)
  • Choose a doctor you feel comfortable talking to. (HHS Five Steps)
  • Ask your doctor about the specialized training and experience that qualifies him or her to treat your illness. (JCAHO Speak Up)

Obviously a move away from the "do as I say" school of "telling people what's good for them" medicine. For example, the relationship-centered model of healthcare practice employed by the Pursuing Perfection Program Team at Whatcom County, Washington, calls for clinical care specialists to fulfill roles as navigators, translators, coaches and lifeguards for chronically ill patients.

As they'll tell you out in Whatcom County, and as we've said here, these kinds of relationships take time to build. They are constructed on a platform of questioning, listening, conversing, respecting and understanding.

What is needed for patients to become activated — to be advocates for their own safe care and treatment? Judith Hibbard, Dr.P.H., professor of health policy, Department of Planning, Public Policy & Management, University of Oregon, is one of the developers of the Patient Activation Measure (PAM). PAM is used to evaluate interventions aimed at engaging patients in their care and to match the level and type of care provided a patient to the patient's ability to manage his or her own care. She makes these points:
  • Patients at first don't think patient safety is their job. One barrier to proactive patient behavior regarding their own safety is that people might not feel confident questioning a doctor. There are norms against this, against questioning authority. It would help if clinicians understood this and were more proactive in engaging patients as partners in their care. No matter how engaged, it is still hard to ask about things like, "Did you wash your hands?"
  • Different patients will be motivated to different degrees. Some people don't feel capable of speaking up, they fear the consequences, or don't know how.
  • The public in general holds a mistaken belief in the consistent high quality of service delivered. Very serious quality gaps in the system that have been documented are not well known by the public. Therefore, there is little motivation to get involved in patient safety.
  • The Patient Activation Measure determines, through a series of questions

asked to patients, the level of knowledge, skill and confidence they possess to become an active collaborator in their own care. For example, a patient is presented with this statement: "When all is said and done, I am the person responsible for managing my health condition." They can strongly disagree, disagree, agree, or strongly agree. Patient activation may be a necessary component of patient-safety and quality improvement programs.

Ten Tips to Activate Patients

Here are ten strategies to help activate patient participation. These go beyond behaviors and involve internal thinking, beliefs, or feeling states. We begin with three guidelines derived from social learning theory: self-efficacy, response-efficacy, and outcome-expectancy.[19] These are critical for overcoming a patient's fear of incompetence and doubt about getting involved.

Elevate self-efficacy

Self-efficacy reflects a "can do" attitude. It refers to a person's perception that he or she can organize and execute, particularly in the case of outpatient care, the instructions necessary to help self-manage their own treatment. To assess whether self-efficacy is sufficient, ask the question, "Do you believe you can do this?" If the answer is "no," then ask, "What would it take to convince you that you can attain the goal?"

Enhance response-efficacy

Response-efficacy refers, again in terms of patient engagement, to one's belief a certain course of treatment, or perhaps a lifestyle change involving diet, alcohol, or smoking, will actually produce the desired outcome. It's not enough to know what to do and have the confidence to do it. You must believe the treatment will work. Will it improve my health?

Sell outcome-expectancy

Outcome-expectancy means a patient believes the effect of participating, of self-monitoring one's own blood pressure, for example, or taking medication as scheduled will produce worthwhile consequences.

This is where you can run into resistance. You can build that "can do" attitude and sell the soundness of a treatment strategy to improve health, but the patient still might not participate. Why? Perhaps the consequence — say losing weight or beginning an exercise regimen — doesn't seem important enough to justify the extra effort and inconvenience. Perhaps the patient has been there, done that — lost weight or started exercise programs before, only to gain back the weight or lose steam with exercise.

What do you do? Often health professionals point to outcome evidence, such as statistics showing the positive benefits of exercise. But these numbers are too abstract, too remote. The consequence a patient can best relate to is an

Case study   *Coaching for patient self-management*

Nancy Stothart, R.N., is a clinical care specialist for the Pursuing Perfection Program in Whatcom County, Bellingham, Washington, and an employee of the Family Care Network, a multi-site family practice group.

I have 34 people under my care. Their illnesses include diabetes, heart failure, chronic pain, mental illness, Parkinson's disease, immune deficiency disorder, and other chronic conditions. The goal is to help patients self-manage their condition and bridge the gaps in the healthcare system to improve their health and quality of life.

I meet with patients wherever it works for them. I visit them at their homes, in the hospital as an inpatient or the emergency department, meet them at their doctors' offices, or at their work. The patient, and how well they're doing, drives the frequency of contact. Some I might call or see once a week or two or three times a week. If they self-manage well and are stable then it may be every month or two. I intervene proactively when something is not working to prevent worsening of their condition.

Chronic conditions are challenging to manage. A diabetes patient I work with had consistently high blood sugars. He had a hard time with his diet. He asked if I could talk to him every day to discuss his blood sugars and diet and help him adjust his insulin per his doctor's directions. After seven weeks his A1C went from 11 to 7. Through frequent contact and support he "got it" and understands how to manage his own care. Support and coaching help patients make and maintain changes.

Patients feel the healthcare system doesn't have the time to listen or care about them. Relationship-based care is more effective and satisfying. We've got it in our heads it takes too much time to develop rapport with people. In our model, patient-centered means the patient is always in focus. Partnerships with patients help them better manage their health. But to help you must understand why the patient is acting the way he or she is.

Say a man has heart disease and won't stop smoking. The doctor might say the patient is "non-compliant." But when asking the patient what they are concerned about, you learn that due to illness he is unable to work and he has no income and is in danger of becoming homeless, and he says, "I need a job because it's really important to me to take care of my child." Smoking is not something he can address until the other stressors in his life are addressed.

Instead of telling people what to do — "Stop smoking" — we start with where the patient is. A lot of us in healthcare think, "If we tell them, they'll do it." Then we get frustrated when they don't do it. Many times they don't understand what they have or what the doctor wants them to do. There is a gap in what they understand.

Sometimes we help patients by interpreting or translating the exchange with the doctor. The doctor might ask a question and not get an answer that relates to what they asked. We rephrase the question and then the patient understands and can answer it. We start with what the patient wants.

The patient-physician interaction can be fraught with misunderstanding. There is a gap in communication. A lot of what we do is fill in the gaps. A patient may have high blood pressure that needs treatment, but the doctor believes the patient doesn't want to go on another medication, "It's expensive and makes them feel crummy." But when the patient understands the risk of stroke or heart attack, they say, "Give it to me." A lot of times I'll hear the patient say, "No one ever told me that."

Our program improves a patient's quality of life. They feel more in control and able to manage their condition. We have also found money is saved through reduced visits to physicians, emergency rooms, and fewer hospital admissions. But most payers would not reimburse us for what we're doing. The healthcare payment structure must change for that to happen.

(The Whatcom County Program was started by a grant funded by the Robert Wood Johnson Foundation. It is a community project partnering with patients, a family practice group, a cardiology group, a hospital and its senior clinic, a community health clinic, and a community-supported healthcare intranet.)

individual one — a personal report of another patient with a similar medical condition who claims the benefits were well worth the treatment costs.

Encourage testimonies

Listeners can relate to an individual's story and put themselves in the same situation. A personal account of a health problem that could have been prevented by certain behaviors is a powerful motivator. So is an anecdote about someone whose health improved by making certain changes in her behavior.

If you want to follow this strategy, your task is to devise a way for patients to network with each other so they can open up and speak frankly about their challenges, frustrations and past experiences. They support each other by owning up to things they could have done to take better care of themselves. Hospital support groups are one model for these types of exchanges.

Let's be clear: We're not talking about shifting the primary responsibility for treatment from caregivers to the patient. Be on the lookout for signs patients are perceiving such a shift. You can alleviate these kinds of concerns by following the next strategy.

Build trust

You're not going to activate, motivate or otherwise involve a patient with a "command and control" mindset typified by writing out instructions and expecting them to be followed. Patients will open up and trust those in charge of their treatment process when they feel part of the process, not merely an "order-taker."

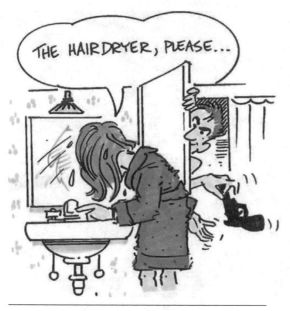

"If you don't know why we're pushing 'patient-centered' medicine you obviously haven't been in a hospital lately," says the senior director for patient safety at a 400-bed hospital in the Midwest. "As a patient you're not at the center, you're not in control. You don't have an advocate usually, and you're not communicated to in a decent way." The next two strategies help build trust with patients:

Blind trust can be hazardous.

Put principles before procedures

When people are educated about their treatment options and the rationale behind the choice to go with one, they can begin to get comfortable with what they must do to make the treatment work. Remember, people are more likely to accept and follow instructions they understand, and have a chance to give input or feedback on. The treatment option chosen becomes "the best way to do it" rather than "an order I must obey."

Customize your process

Don't build your patient engagement efforts around off-the-shelf handouts you distribute without elaboration and simply expect patients to follow. Your customers, to put it in business terms, want more personalized service.

Yes, there are certain things patients must do. Mandates or directions are unavoidable at times. But in delivering your "service" to patients, try a blend of confidence and openness. Of course it's important to project confidence in a selected course of action, and a degree of uncertainty is natural if outcome prospects are questionable. But leave room for the patient to be mindful, resourceful, and self-motivated. This freedom from control boosts trust, and in turn leads to more involvement. Dr. Hibbard's Patient Activation Measure is one method for determining how knowledgeable, confident and motivated a patient is, and how much "space" you can give them to self-manage.

Cultivate self-persuasion & self-accountability

Choice, ownership, and trust contribute to self-accountability — a necessity for patients taking a more active role in their care. Especially when patients are not under direct supervision and care, they need to hold themselves accountable to follow instructions relating to diet, testing or monitoring, and medication, for example. This often requires a significant amount of self-persuasion or self-discipline.

Condescending lectures or incentives for lifestyle changes (such as those offered by some employers for wellness activities) are often not the best motivators. Research has shown the more external justification a person feels for a certain activity or behavior, the less internal justification or self-accountability the individual develops.[20]

Use the hypocrisy effect

Instead of intimidiation or incentives, try this technique: First, obtain the patient's commitment that he or she will perform designated healthy behavior(s). Getting the patient to "buy-in" in front of family members will tend to strengthen this commitment. Then ask for a list of personal at-risk actions that are inconsistent with the desired healthy behavior. You're stirring up tension between words (the commitment) and deeds (prior behavior), which in turn increases self-persuasion and self-accountability to live up to the commitment.

By getting people to experience hypocrisy (or feelings of inconsistency), they are more likely to perform the healthy behavior when alone in order to reduce the tension. The need to be consistent in word and deed can have broad impact, as reflected in the final guideline we give you for fueling patient participation.

Promote systems thinking

Yes, that's right. Bring systems thinking into patient engagement. Here's what we mean: When a patient chooses to change a behavior, they adjust their attitudes and beliefs to be consistent with their actions. This change in attitude can influence more behavior change — a spiraling, reciprocal interdependency between outward actions and inward feelings. This is how small changes in behavior and attitude can eventually lead to a patient's strong personal commitment and full involvement in the process of healthcare.

One benefit of this sort of systems thinking for patient-centered medicine is that it shows the patient the variety of internal and external factors that can affect his or her ability to self-manage part of their own care. It relieves them of blame or guilt over being a "bad patient." Instead, being enlightened to the bigger picture provides direction for self-persuasion and self-accountability.

FAQ *How do you build cohesive teams in healthcare?*

Healthcare teams can be more difficult to pull together than teams in an airline cockpit or factory production shift. Care-giving often involves many specialists who come and go, floaters and part-timers, and physicians on-site for only short periods each day. So how do you build cohesive teams in healthcare?

The foundation already exists. From the time a patient is admitted to a healthcare setting until he or she is discharged, various types of teamwork occur all along the way. The special challenge in a healthcare setting is the members of diverse teams continually change. Thus, individual members do not know who to expect or what to expect. This requires a special commitment to interdependency among healthcare professionals.

Trust is essential. More specifically, it is critical to trust the intentions and the abilities of the team members, even though membership is fluid. How do you build such trust? We recommend considering the following five words, each beginning with the letter "C" and each implying particular behaviors:

*1. **Communication** – It is essential to exchange information and opinions among team members. Open and frank communication is needed throughout the process of teamwork.*

*2. **Candor** – The communication between team members needs to be straightforward and frank, and free from prejudice.*

*3. **Caring** – Team members need to show they care, and this is obvious among healthcare workers. Indeed, the word "care" is part of their job title.*

*4. **Consistency** – Team members need to be consistent, meaning when they say they will do something they do it. And behaviors need to be consistent with values. If patient care is a value then a person's behaviors should reflect that.*

*5. **Consensus** – Team members attempt to reach consensus on issues. For example, instead of voting to decide whose opinion should win, the group should take more time to reach unanimity. There should be no minority opinion, but only a group consensus.*

Finally, trust and teamwork is facilitated by "positive gossip." Specifically, people need to talk about the strengths and positive attributes of others. This enables interpersonal recognition and appreciation of team members' talents and value to the team.

Unfortunately, negative gossip is more popular than positive gossip. When someone shares something negative about another person to you, don't you wonder, "What does this person say about me behind my back?" Consider how this destroys trust and inhibits constructive teamwork. But also consider how easy it is to stop negative backstabbing. Simply do not pay attention to such conversation. When someone starts to backstab, simply say, "I am not interested. Do you have something positive to say about this person?"

CHAPTER 4 *Thinking*

In this chapter you'll learn:

How do you respond to the thinking that errors are inevitable?

How do you move mindsets from worry and anxiety over safety to personal control and optimism?

1 How we talk ourselves into taking personal responsibility

What are your personal reasons for choosing safe behavior?

How often do you buckle your safety belt automatically, without thinking?

Most people will say they buckle-up for safety out of habit. That's good, but not great. It would be better to think about what you're doing while fastening your safety belt.

We're talking about "conscious competence," which is usually better than "unconscious competence," like habitually buckling up. This is especially true when it comes to safety-related behavior.

You see, the conscious rationale we provide ourselves for performing safe behavior is determined by our thinking — our non-stop, 24/7 self-talk or internal verbal behavior. To prevent medical errors and increase the quality of patient care, it's important to tell yourself what you are doing when you perform a patient-safety-related behavior.

For the safety-belt example, you would use self-talk that acknowledges the behavior — "I'm buckling up for safety."

When safe behavior is accomplished for positive consequences — such as patient welfare — it helps to also verbalize the rationale for the behavior. What are your personal reasons for choosing safe behavior?

For example, when you report an event involving a medical error, you might say to yourself, "Reporting errors makes a difference. Reporting is a critical information source for creating a safe healthcare environment."

When it comes to adhering to hand-hygiene protocol, your self-talk might be: "Clean hands are critical to preventing cross-transmission and reducing healthcare-associated infections."

In both of these examples, it's possible your action is not self-directed (as when buckling your safety belt) but rather other-directed. In other words, you might be filing an incident report or washing your hands because it's a matter of policy or it's a requirement. If your safe behavior is other-directed, your self-talk should not include the external "controls" influencing your behavior. Until you can give a self-directed rationale, you should only tell yourself you are performing the behavior. Here's why:

Self-persuasion: Your self-talk influences self-persuasion, which in turn enhances self-accountability for patient safety. Indeed, we hold ourselves accountable by talking to ourselves. The kind of self-talk that builds our self-accountability or responsibility for patient safety is not going to be predicated on pleasing others.

Indeed, we can be motivated by both outside and inside controls. But the more our behavior is directed and motivated from within ourselves, the more apt we are to perform the behavior when alone and only accountable to ourselves. This is essential for the many times caregivers work alone.

Self-talk is the tool for putting ourselves in this motivated, self-accountable frame of mind. We talk ourselves into feeling personally responsible.

Now some situations facilitate this thinking; some do not. In general, self-accountability thinking decreases as the degree of external negative control increases. Severe threats and strong enforcement do this. Then people's perception of personal choice decreases. This could explain why numerous caregivers do not hold themselves accountable for reporting medical errors. In one study, reasons given for not reporting included "concerned about being blamed or judged incompetent" and "concerned about implicating others"[1] — both external negative influences.

Self-talk, self-perception and self-accountability are influenced by our behavior. The more a behavior aligns with our sense of who we are — our core values — the more we will feel accountable for that behavior.

So, what kind of person are you? Do you hold patient safety as a core value? How do you know?

Our behavior defines us. But there are exceptions. When we believe our behavior is controlled entirely by external factors, we do not view that behavior as a reflection of who we are.

When we perceive our behavior as self-directed, we use the behavior to define our attitudes and values. In other words, behaviors we choose to perform provide information for our self-perception and self-talk. These behaviors are certainly motivated by expected consequences, both intrinsic and extrinsic. The key is to perceive some degree of choice, and perception of choice is stifled by enforcement or negative reinforcement contingencies. For example, we perceive minimal choice when we fail to report an incident out of fear of blame or getting someone else in trouble.

Self-perception and values: Self-directed behavior informs our self-perception and our core values. And our self-perception and personal values influence our behavior. We strive for our behavior to be consistent with our values, and vice versa. When we perceive an inconsistency between behavior and the values that define us, we experience tension or "cognitive dissonance" (the academic label used by the many social psychologists who researched this phenomenon)[2]. We direct our self-talk to reduce this tension.

"I know hand hygiene is important, but I just don't have the time. Why don't they make the wash stations more accessible?"

The rationale we provide ourselves for performing — or neglecting — safe behavior determines whether we feel self-accountable and will continue to perform that behavior in the absence of an external accountability system. Using the self-talk cited above, a person would not be likely to clean up before patient contact because they've removed self-accountability. They've shifted accountability to the system, including time pressures and inadequate placement of wash stations.

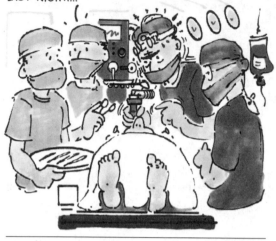

THIS EXTREMELY DANGEROUS BRAIN SURGERY IS AIDED BY THE MOST HIGH-TECH, STATE-OF-THE-ART PROBING DEVICE EVER ENGINEERED... BUT YOU KNOW THE SURGEON TOTALED HIS PORSCHE LAST NIGHT....

Irrelevant self-talk can be dangerous.

We hope you see the critical importance of our thinking and self-talk. People-Based Patient Safety™ teaches the kind of thinking needed to develop self-accountability, as well as the kinds of environmental and management conditions and systems needed to promote and support self-accountability thinking in healthcare.

In Chapter 4, we discuss common barriers in healthcare that interfere with self-talk and self-accountability, and we offer tools and techniques to develop a positive, persuasive mental script.

2 Antidotes for "just not thinking"

Use self-talk to both prepare for a task and stay mindful during a task

How many patient injuries or near-injuries occur because people were "just not thinking"? How often do caregivers get into a work routine involving a sequence of behaviors performed unconsciously? Operating on "automatic pilot" can lead to startling, and potentially harmful results. For example:

During a hospital stay, an elderly gentleman developed a deep vein thrombosis. When he was discharged, he received enoxaparin for self-injection at home, along with other medications. Before leaving the hospital, he received written information sheets covering his medications and counseling from a nurse and a pharmacist.

Several days later, the patient called the primary care triage nurse and explained he had been discharged with a bag of medications and some injections, but he couldn't administer them because he can't read the instructions. After retrieving his chart, the triage nurse discovered the patient is blind, and also that he lives alone.[3]

Could it be that discharging a patient is one of those daily regimens that caregivers move through with little thought, alertness, or creativity? The more mundane and commonplace the activity, the more likely a person will use an unconscious script to guide behavior — with an accompanying lack of awareness. In this case, the nurse and pharmacist were unaware their patient was blind.

Mindless activity is fine if habitual behaviors are safe and the routine is stable, without variance. But what if something unexpected and unusual happens, such as a blind patient waiting to be discharged? Our lack of awareness, or our mindlessness at the time, can prevent prompt reaction. That's what occurred with the blind patient. Without even realizing it, mindless work practice put the patient at risk for harm.

So how do we become more mindful of behavioral routines that could lead to patient harm?

One method you can use to monitor and control your self-talk is through a mental checklist. That's a list in your mind of critical actions you need to take to complete a task safely.

We can control our self-talk with a mental checklist that reminds us of critical safe actions, or thoughts that help us stay in the moment. It's called a mental checklist because it isn't written down. We merely think it up. It's one way to remember details when the environment is full of interruptions and distractions. We repeat a mental checklist to ourselves in order to stay mindful of what we're doing.

We're not talking about cheap trick pop psychology here. This isn't a matter of pasting positive affirmation notes on your mirror to read in the morning, or writing mental motivational messages to pull out of your pocket during the day. This is a behavioral checklist we keep in our awareness through specific self-talk. Before we talk to ourselves to remind us what to do, and when we are acting, we tell ourselves what we are doing. Thus, we use self-talk to both prepare for a task and stay mindful during a task.

Mental checklist: One of the most effective checklists is the simple universal checklist called S.T.A.R.T. that we described in Chapter 2 on Acting. You'll recall the steps:

STOP before every procedure. Put all action on pause for one to five seconds.

Then THINK about what needs to be done, critical safe action by critical safe action. Finally, imagine the successful outcome.

Take an active role in your imagination. Don't just see it as if you're watching an inner movie. Feel yourself actually there, as if it were really happening. Imagine each step you need to take.

Then — and only then — complete the next three steps in the S.T.A.R.T. process: ACT, REVIEW and TRACK what you've just done.

Research also shows the benefits of informal verbal persuasion. In one study,[4] 60 male, undergraduate students at a university in Greece were divided randomly into one control and two self-talk groups. These students were asked to shoot basketballs for three minutes, from a 14.75-foot distance to the hoop, using five different positions on the perimeter of an arc. Initially, members of all three groups received instructions to complete as many successful shots as possible in a three-minute time span.

After this three-minute trial, all 60 shooters rested for 20 minutes. During the 20-minute break, members of the two self-talk groups received in private new, specific instructions. Students in one self-talk group were asked to utter the cue-word "relax" prior to each shot at the hoop, while individuals in the second group were requested to repeat the word "fast" before every attempt at the goal. Control-group players received the same instructions given before the test trial ("execute as many successful shots as possible").

The outcome: the "relax" group sank significantly more shots in the third trial, compared to the "fast" and control subjects.

This study also demonstrates the importance of making sure your self-talk is task-relevant. "Relax" is a reassuring directive often employed by athletes and recommended by sports psychologists; it is a term which often tends to improve concentration, while slowing athletes' movements down slightly. "Fast" is a self-talk injunction which may well lead to greater quickness, perhaps at the expense of optimal movement, effectiveness and accuracy.[5]

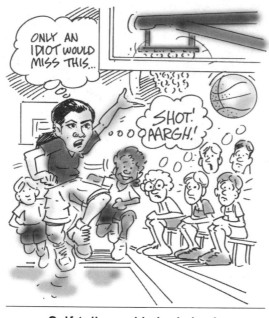

Self-talk can hinder behavior.

Peer observations: Here's another consideration: Optimal mindfulness during complex activities is not something you achieve on your own. It requires support of others. In the sports psychology example above, you can see the importance of coaching. In the workplace, group consciousness-raising can be developed through an observation and feedback process, such as described in Chapter 2 on Acting.

Imagine one caregiver approaching another who is hard at work and asking, "Is this a good time for a behavioral audit?" Whether the answer is "yes" or "no," some amount of safety mindfulness is raised. Now consider the impact of the actual observation process on task-specific awareness. After volunteering to be observed, the worker is now mindful of every aspect of his or her job. The employee not only thinks about the specific items on the critical behavior checklist, but tries to be cognizant of every possible safety-related behavior of the task.

The positive effect of observation on mindfulness was noted in a study of hand-hygiene practices at an acute care hospital in Switzerland.[6] Although the observer in this case was as unobtrusive as possible, researchers stated "aware-ness of being observed was strongly associated with adherence" (to hand-hygiene recommendations).

Mindfulness at its best is initiated by an observation process that includes several key elements: communication is open and direct, the focus is on behaviors, and the observation is only conducted with permission. This helps to build the proper context — an atmosphere of interpersonal trust and actively caring.

The individual feedback portion of this behavioral coaching process is certainly important. It supports the safe decisions a coworker makes, and provides an opportunity to improve job safety. Feedback also makes both employees, the observed and the observer, more mindful of the many environmental and behavioral facets of the work process that could cause personal injury.

A few words about observation etiquette: Unannounced observations might give a more realistic picture of the at-risk behaviors occurring while someone works, but such audits risk reducing interpersonal trust and giving the impression that People-Based Patient Safety™ is a negative "gotcha" program.

From a behavior-change perspective, observations without permission cannot raise safety mindfulness. It's likely the mindfulness developed and increased from an open and voluntary behavioral observation process is critical for behavior change and patient welfare. To get the best from such a process we need to be mindful of what it takes to develop and maintain an atmosphere of interpersonal trust and "actively caring."

Group exercise: Here's an idea for promoting mindfulness at a patient-safety meeting. Pass out a raisin to everyone at the meeting and ask participants to place the raisin on their tongues. Then, request each person to close their eyes and very slowly chew on their raisin, attending to every aspect of the raisin: its shape, texture, and taste. The aim is to become aware — or mindful — of every aspect of this single raisin-eating experience.

Psychotherapists use this raisin-eating exercise to help people reduce their adverse reaction to stressors. In fact, this is a common stress-reduction exercise for heart patients who need to decrease their blood pressure. So you might use the raisin exercise as a stress-reduction technique. By having participants slow down to experience the process of eating a single raisin, they learn how to intentionally slow down their thinking and body processes and put themselves in a state of relaxation.

This can be a thoughtful interlude for caregivers who make hundreds of decisions every day, in the estimate of David W. Bates, M.D., chief of the Division of General Medicine at Brigham and Women's Hospital in Boston, Massachusetts, and professor of medicine at Harvard Medical School. "It is hard for us to slow down decision-making," he says.

3 How to develop self-accountability for patient safety

Take an informal mental inventory of your actions

What was she thinking?

A nurse entered the hospital room of a 67-year-old man, still groggy from anesthesia two hours after he had undergone a laminectomy. It's time to administer his clonazepam, the nurse announced. The patient began to take his medicine, but his daughter, who happened to be a nurse, interrupted, saying she didn't think he should be receiving clonazepam. She asked the nurse to double check. The nurse returned after checking and asked, "Aren't you Mr. X?" "No, I am Mr. J," the patient answered.[7]

When we work alone, like the nurse above, we need to hold ourselves accountable for patient safety, and that requires a sense of personal responsibility. How do we do it?

Interpersonal safety coaching isn't relevant here. But the very essence of People-Based Patient Safety™ is a process we call safety self-management. It's a way of getting caregivers to act themselves into feeling more personally responsible for patient safety when no one is around to hold them accountable. Here are ten techniques for keeping lone caregivers self-accountable for patient safety.

1) Observe your own behavior

Develop a checklist (it could be written or rehearsed mentally as described above) with a number of critical patient-safety-related behaviors to observe while you work. Every time an opportunity for a particular target behavior occurs, simply judge whether your behavior was safe or at-risk. At the end of a shift, total up the approximate number of safe and at-risk occurrences for each behavior to roughly calculate a "percent safe" score.

In industry, we've seen many cases where this self-assessment is a formal, written process completed on a daily and weekly basis by individuals. This formal approach allows you to chart personal performance on a graph to track daily or weekly fluctuation. Recording and charting "percent safe" scores will significantly improve safety because it gets you involved; you become accountable to yourself.

We realize you are constantly interrupted during the day and might not have the opportunity to write down and chart safe or at-risk behaviors relating to patient safety. Still, an informal mental inventory of your actions will help you discover that a few at-risk behaviors occur more frequently. They become the targets of your self-management process.

2) Analyze the activator-behavior-consequence sequence

As explained in Chapter 2, a key principle of People-Based Patient Safety™ is actions are directed by activators or events preceding behavior, and are motivated by consequences or events following behavior. During your self-observation process, note activators and consequences relevant to critical behaviors for patient safety. You might be able to remove activators or consequences that encourage or reward at-risk behavior. Or you might be able to add activators or consequences to increase certain safe behaviors.

3) Take control of activators

Posters, signs, and other reminders are the most popular activators for safety. But only a small portion of the many activators we see each day actually influences our behavior. We're often in a state of information overload where we either don't notice or ignore many activators. Still, we can place a few activators in strategic locations as reminders. Or we can tell ourselves to pay attention to certain activators that encourage safe behavior or discourage particular at-risk behavior.

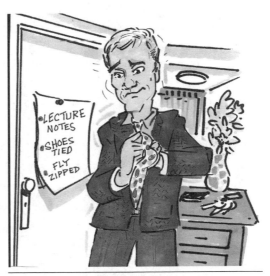

Strategically placed activators can be critical reminders.

4) Cue your own performance

If you say to yourself, "I report medical errors to set an example. My behavior could influence anyone who sees me, especially a department member, and I don't want anyone to think I'm irresponsible about medical error," you're likely to report incidents. Notice that this self-dialogue includes specific instructions, and expresses a belief about the value of setting an example that provides a strong rationale for acting on behalf of patient safety. Note, too, how your beliefs influence your perception or interpretation of personal events.

Observations can shed light on your true beliefs. What does it say about your patient-safety beliefs if you realize you forgot to give a child his morning dose of seizure medication, but decided not to report the error because the order was finally given three hours late, and the child had no apparent ill effects? After all, you tell yourself, it was only a minor close call. You might find you're not being entirely truthful when you say patient safety is one of your core values. Perhaps you'll discover an inconsistency between something you value and the way you act. This can motivate you to make a behavioral adjustment.

5) Reward yourself

Research shows people who reward themselves are more likely to sustain a self-management process and improve their own performance.[8] Three factors determine the effect of these rewards: selection, delivery, and timing.

First, personalize your reward. The possibilities are endless. We could be talking about opportunities to exercise, eat certain foods, spend money, attend an entertaining event, watch television, or say to yourself with pride, "I did it." It's a matter of giving yourself an opportunity to do something enjoyable after you've done something less fun but important for patient safety, and personal improvement.

Base your rewards on specific behavior, not affirmations or good intentions. Observe your behavior systematically and reward yourself according to criteria you define. The reward should come as soon as possible after the target behavior occurs.

6) Set SMART goals

Rewards should be directed at a "SMART" goal — one that is Specific, Motivational, Achievable, Relevant, and Trackable as explained in Chapter 2. At first, give yourself rewards to recognize small steps of progress toward the goal. During the early stages of self-management, it's often useful to reward yourself for just participating in the process. In one self-management project, for example, a woman rewarded herself by adding $1 to her vacation fund each day she completed her self-observing and recording. Later she rewarded herself only when her target behavior improved. Continuous improvement occurred by successively requiring more behavior for the $1 reward. Eventually, one SMART goal was reached, and then another, more challenging SMART goal was set.

7) Chart progress and celebrate your success

SMART goals are potent self-motivators because you state them in a way that enables you to objectively monitor personal progress. When a specified level of achievement is reached, you should celebrate. It can be a personal celebration, perhaps as simple as giving yourself a pat on the back. Better yet, give yourself one of those opportunities for some personal pleasure.

Involving other people in your celebration is even more effective. Tell others about your efforts to become more personally responsible for patient safety and invite them to help you celebrate. If you tell others you intend to improve certain target behaviors, the likelihood you will actually improve increases.

8) Make a commitment

When you publicly commit to doing something, you create both internal and external pressures to follow through. So make a formal commitment to improve your actions and attitudes relating to patient safety and reducing medical error. You can do this by:

• Signing and publicly displaying a simple pledge card that states your intention to participate in a self-management process and reach a certain patient-safety-improvement goal.

• Signing an interpersonal contract with a friend or coworker that specifies the patient-safety-related behavior you wish to improve and includes a brief outline of your plan for accomplishing this goal.

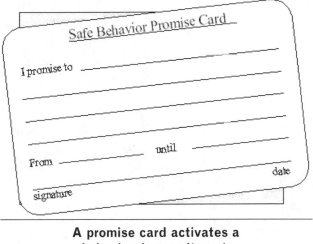

A promise card activates a behavioral commitment.

There are numerous benefits of involving others in your self-management work. They can hold you accountable to initiate and maintain your efforts, and encourage you to keep going. Plus, they can make a celebration more reinforcing.

9) Enlist social support

You can get invaluable encouragement from a work culture where caregivers trust each other's abilities and intentions, as well as feel a sense of belonging and interdependency. You'll be more willing to accept personal responsibility for patient safety when you believe your coworkers genuinely want you to improve.

When you take control of monitoring and managing your actions and attitudes for patient safety, you create a supportive social context for yourself. You look for others who might appreciate your personal commitment, and enlist support from supervisors, coworkers, friends, or family members who you know care.

10) Use imagery

Mental imagery is using your "mind's eye" to picture situations without actually being there. It's a way to anticipate and prepare for events. It can be used to direct behavior (as an activator), and to motivate behavior (as a consequence). In fact, mental imagery can be very useful in increasing personal responsibility for safety in the absence of a formal self-management project. In the next section, we'll talk more about this safety improvement technique.

4 How to use your mind's eye to prevent errors

Use mental imagery to rehearse the job

Mental imagery is using our "mind's eye" to picture situations without actually being there. It's something we do every day.

When we look forward to a particular event, for instance, we use imagery. Picturing pleasant consequences can lead to excitement, even an emotional high. In contrast, imagining negative outcomes can evoke fear. In fact, one of the most effective ways to relieve distress or anxiety is to visualize your-self in a serene and relaxing setting (like lying on a sandy beach and hearing the calming rhythm of the ocean waves, and feeling the warm sun and cool breeze).

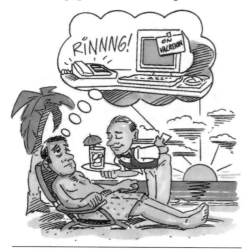

A mental image can ruin a vacation.

When you think about the behav-ioral steps or procedures needed to complete a task, you're using mental images to rehearse the job. Before their performances, athletes practice their sport mentally, actors run through their lines and stage positions in their mind's eye, surgeons mentally rehearse the steps of a complex operation, and musicians imagine playing or singing the right notes on key and on time. Public speakers often practice their lines mentally just prior to actual delivery.

Research has shown significant benefits of mental rehearsal, whether prac-ticing an athletic skill, an occupational task, or a script of dialogue.[9] It's not clear whether the mental rehearsal actually strengthens the correct behavior or merely increases personal motivation to perform at a higher level. We don't know why mental rehearsal improves performance, only that it does. The more vividly people imagine themselves performing desired behaviors, the greater the beneficial impact of this technique on actual performance. Now what does all this mean for keeping patients from harm?

Making the connection

We could not find any research on the effects of imagery on safety-related behavior. But given the variety of performance behaviors that have benefited from this practice, it's obviously a useful tool to prevent injury. We can mentally rehearse images to anticipate and prepare for tasks. Imagery can direct our behavior (as an activator) or motivate our behavior (as a consequence). For safety self-management you can use imagery to:

- Clarify your safety goals
- Enhance your motivation to choose the safest behavior
- Build your self-efficacy, personal control, or optimism
- Rehearse safe acts and actively caring behaviors
- Reward yourself for success at self-management

It's often more useful to create a mental picture of positive consequences resulting from your safe actions. Focusing on positive outcomes can increase your confidence in being successful, as well as increase your desire to reach your goals.

Here's how to use mental imagery to manage your own safety:

- See yourself performing the appropriate safe behavior with ease and convenience — checking for two patient identifiers, reading back a prescription order using phonetic pronunciation, executing a hand-off following SBAR protocol.
- Visualize avoiding specific negative consequences with the safe behavior — a harmed patient, a grieving family.
- Imagine feelings of accomplishment following the safe behavior.
- Take an active rather than passive perspective.
- Share your imagery with others to get support and perhaps increase their safe behavior.

It's important to be active in your image. Don't sit back and watch a movie starring yourself. Imagine yourself acting within the complete activator-behavior- consequence framework. First, see the activators in the situation which cue your desired behavior. Then visualize yourself actually performing the safe acts. Finally, imagine positive feelings from setting the safe example and acknowledging safety as a value.

Share your motivating imagery with others, too. In fact, one reason personal stories of patient injuries or close calls are powerful motivators is because listeners can get a powerful mental image. They can readily visualize the patient in the precarious situation described, especially if the presenter gives a passionate and realistic delivery. Even more motivating are times when listeners imagine themselves or a family member in the place of the patient. Of course, it's essential to focus on the specific behaviors that can be performed to avoid the harm to patients or close calls discussed.

The right kind of mental imagery can motivate us to assume increased personal responsibility for the safety of patients. We can rehearse mentally the safe way to complete a hand-off or identify a patient, and thus increase the likelihood the task will be accomplished both safely and efficiently.

We can also teach others how to use mental pictures to prevent risk and patient harm. Let's encourage personal testimonials of negative events or close calls that could have been prevented by certain action. We need to hold ourselves accountable for using and teaching this effective patient-safety self-management technique.

5 The motivating power of choice
Be mindful of your self-talk

By now, you know we always have a choice of which action to take. Did you know we also have a choice what to think? Sometimes we're not aware of our choices unless we're mindful of self-talk. Positive self-talk empowers us to do what we can to keep patients out of harm's way. These basic beliefs are key to empowerment — and they exemplify positive self-talk:

• "I can do it and it will work."
• "I'm motivated to make it work."
• "I can and want to do it."
• "I want to make a difference."

Positive self-talk motivates us to think about safety. Positive self-talk can also bolster our confidence — and when we're more confident, we're more apt to do the right thing.

The alternative, negative self-talk, is subversive:

• "I'm a nervous wreck."
• "I don't see anyone else scrubbing up."
• "It's not my job to be a role model in this department."
• "No one else is speaking up. They must know what they're doing."

If you reflect on your own life circumstances, you'll quickly see how a sense of choice or personal control makes you more motivated, involved, and committed. We've all experienced the pleasure of having alternatives to choose from and feeling in control of those factors critical for success. And when it comes to how we think, we certainly have alternatives to choose from.

Of course we're not always in control of critical events or ongoing circumstances that affect our thoughts, especially in the unpredictable world of healthcare. The message is clear to system managers. Give people the power to choose patient-safety procedures consistent with the right principles, and the result will be perceptions of personal control and self-effectiveness. This might require changes in leadership style:

• Relinquishing some top-down control
• Abandoning a desire for the "quick fix"
• Switching from focusing on outcomes to recognizing process achievements
• Giving people opportunities to choose, evaluate, and refine their means to achieve the ends.

But what can be done for physicians and nurses who feel a loss of control, autonomy and authority when told to use checklists, scripts or follow mandatory procedures? How can they overcome feelings of loss of power and control?

The challenge is to convince caregivers that the use of certain tools (behavioral checklists, environmental audits, job-specific briefings, interpersonal coaching, and process goal-setting) can improve patient safety. Then their involvement in developing the specific protocol for applying these tools will lead to perceptions of personal control and competence. They will feel a sense of empowerment and ownership to use these tools when they believe:

- They can use them effectively.
- The tools will work to improve patient safety.
- The time and inconvenience of using the tools are cost effective.

Development and use of tools to improve patient safety should increase, not decrease the perception of control among healthcare workers. Standardization is only relevant regarding guidelines for using certain patient-safety tools or procedures. The particular process for using these tools is defined by the staff who use them. And it's critical to refine the tools as they are used. Who does this refinement? Staff develops and refines the tools they use for patient safety. This

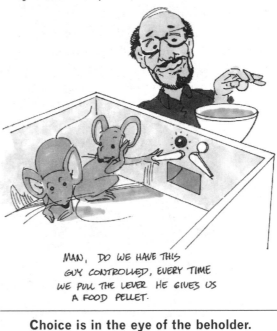

MAN, DO WE HAVE THIS GUY CONTROLLED, EVERY TIME WE PULL THE LEVER HE GIVES US A FOOD PELLET.

Choice is in the eye of the beholder.

is key to developing a sense of personal control and accountability.

Remember, self-talk and self-persuasion will most likely be used by those who have a high internal locus of control.[10] And self-effectiveness will be unpredictable when a situation (or a system) is ambiguous, lacks relevant information, or contains a high degree of uncertainty or poor organization.[11]

6   How to build a supportive belief system
Beliefs contribute to our self-talk

Self-talk can be positive or negative, influencing behavior that can be safe or risky. Self-talk is based on behavior, perceptions, and beliefs — which "can exist with or without evidence that they are accurate" — some which are formed early in life.[12]

Beliefs contribute to our self-talk, which in turn affects our self-efficacy. There is empirical and theoretical support for the assertion that believing you can do something is the first step toward doing it. The academic term for this belief is "self-efficacy," and it has been the topic of many research articles and theoretical proposals. Most notable is Albert Bandura's 1997 book, entitled simply, *Self-Efficacy.*[13] Here, in 604 pages of fine print, the author makes a strong case for self-efficacy being the most central and critical concept in applied psychology. The main features of this concept are self-efficacy, response-efficacy, and outcome-expectancy.

These psychological terms determine whether a person feels empowered. First, when you promote "can do" self-talk toward safety, you're promoting self-efficacy. Numerous studies have shown that people with strong "can do" thinking demonstrate greater ability and motivation to solve problems at work. And they have better health and safety habits.[14]

But it's not enough to convince yourself and others we "can do" patient safety. People must believe their plan for patient safety will be effective. This is called response-efficacy.

Finally, people must believe patient safety is worth the effort. This is outcome-expectancy.

So how do you instill these beliefs to support the kind of self-talk that increases patient care and prevent negative events?

Building skills

First, be patient. It takes training, practice and feedback over time to develop the sense of mastery that usually leads to the belief of self-efficacy.

And please note that self-efficacy is not the same as self-esteem, though these beliefs tend to influence each other. Self-esteem reflects a general sense of self-worth, as in, "I am valuable." Self-efficacy refers to feeling successful or competent at a particular task. Self-esteem remains rather constant across situations. Self-efficacy is task-focused and can vary markedly from one circumstance to another.

Yet even when caregivers have both self-efficacy and adequate skills to execute their patient-safety plan, they won't do it unless they believe their plan will work — response-efficacy.

Proving the payoff

It's not enough to know what to do and have the confidence to do it. You can have the skills and self-efficacy to perform patient-safety coaching, for example, but you will not actually coach on a regular basis unless you believe the coaching process actually improves patient safety. The same holds true for teamwork. A number of healthcare professionals are skeptical of teamwork's benefits. So how do you convince yourself and others that certain patient-safety techniques will pay off?

The most common approach is to use statistics that show significant improvement as a result of a particular safety strategy. But people don't necessarily relate to these numbers. It's better to get more personal when trying to "sell" the value of a patient-safety process to a unit.

Research on risk perception, for example, has shown that people get more concerned or outraged about an issue when individual case studies are used in lieu of group statistics.[15] That's why politicians like to point out specific individuals in their audiences when trying to gain support for a particular issue or plan.

Personal testimonies provide a powerful image. Listeners can relate to a person's story and put themselves in the same situation. Two kinds of testimonies can increase response-efficacy:

A personal account of harm to a patient that could have been prevented by a certain safety technique; and

An anecdote about a patient who avoided harm by a caregiver's use of a particular strategy or safety process.

But is it worth it?

We might believe we can do something for patient safety. We also might believe that what we do will have a positive effect. But we won't get involved unless we also believe the outcome is worth working for.

In patient safety, for example, some people might believe a 90-percent adherence to hand-hygiene recommendations is good enough, given they see very few patients getting infections. The potential gain from the inconvenience of getting that last 10 percent of adherence might seem too small to justify the amount of extra effort required.

Remember, too, the common perception among physicians is that errors are made by someone else.[16] In one study, only 29 percent of physicians reported encountering any medical error in the past year.[17] As a result, the need to participate in a patient-safety effort can seem insignificant.

Consequences keep us going — we've mentioned this many times throughout this book. One of B. F. Skinner's most important legacies is the principle that we motivate ourselves to do or not do something by anticipating what positive consequences we expect to gain from our participation — and/or what negative consequences we expect to avoid.[18]

To build outcome-expectancy — the belief the consequences are worth your effort — we suggest again "selling" with a case study rather than statistics. For example, show the details of a single patient injury that occurred on your floor. Explain how an intervention like the one being taught could have prevented that incident.

Part of your "selling" is to get people to see the bigger picture. Move them away from an individualistic "error-won't-happen-to- me" mindset. You want to develop systems thinkers who take a wider view, and realize some patient somewhere will benefit from large-scale participation in your patient-safety process.

Appeal to frontline caregivers' natural concern and caring for patients. When people see the bigger picture and adopt a "collective community" perspective, they realize their participation in a patient-safety process will even-

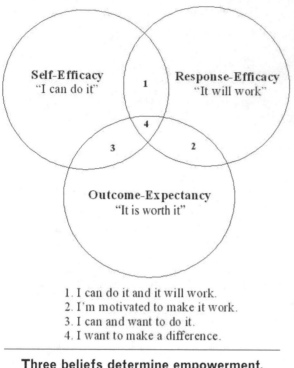

1. I can do it and it will work.
2. I'm motivated to make it work.
3. I can and want to do it.
4. I want to make a difference.

Three beliefs determine empowerment.

tually benefit patients throughout the system. You will find this belief — that it's meaningful to work for the potential benefit of preventing errors and increasing quality care — fuels self-efficacy and response-efficacy.

(We have much more to say about selling patient safety in Chapter 6 — Keeping it Going.)

Pop psychologists and motivational speakers are right; beliefs and self-talk are important in determining success. But we need to go beyond self-affirmation or self-confidence and self-talk to meet the challenges of patient safety. Inspiring the three beliefs we've discussed here — both in yourself and others — defines true empowerment. They are key to maximizing participation, personal responsibility, and success in a patient-safety process.

7   Why feedback is crucial to prevent thinking-related errors

And essential to support mindful, safe decisions

Feedback is certainly important in developing mindfulness. It supports the safe decisions you make, and provides an opportunity to improve patient-safety aspects of a job. Unfortunately, when it comes to matters of mental performance, there is in medicine what Dr. Mark Graber calls "a lack of calibration."[19]"Doctors don't get enough feedback on their performance, and that leads to denial and complacency," he told us in an interview. "They don't realize how many errors they make; there's no appreciation because they get no feedback. A lot of doctors think they're doing just fine."

One calibration tool seldom used today is the autopsy. In the United States, the autopsy rate is now estimated to be less than five percent.[20]

Deprived of such learning tools, "it's amazing how often doctors are correct" in their diagnoses and decision-making, says Dr. Graber.

But physicians aren't alone in lacking feedback. Studies demonstrate a universal tendency to over-estimate our own abilities, and one reason is people in general seldom receive corrective feedback about their behaviors. In our society we remind each other, "If you don't have something nice to say, don't say anything at all."[21] And to make constructive learning even less likely, when people do receive an evaluation, such as a year-end job performance review, seldom is time taken to explain how the evaluation was derived, what specific skills were assessed.

Filling in the feedback void — in healthcare or elsewhere — requires a structured approach and a degree of organization. But please design feedback to be more effective than the customary three-minute performance review. Feedback channels can involve coaching, regular team debriefings, and training classes with critiques on how to maintain situational awareness within a local, perhaps unit-level, environment.

You can also give yourself feedback, by reviewing and reflecting on your use of a formal or informal mental checklist of critical patient-safety actions you should follow, as we described earlier in this chapter.

Expert Q&A   *How I became reflective about safety*

Jeffrey B. Cooper, Ph.D., is a patient-safety pioneer. His 1978 paper, "Preventable Anesthesia Mishaps: A study in human factors," was the first in-depth, scientific look at errors in medicine, based on analysis of 359 errors. Today, Dr. Cooper is director of biomedical engineering for Partners HealthCare System, Inc.; associate professor of anesthesia at Harvard Medical School; and executive director of the Center for Medical Simulation in Cambridge, Massachusetts.

Q *You've mentioned in interviews that you've spent a lot of time over the years analyzing your own errors. Is this because you're an engineer by training, and engineers, as you suggest, are schooled to think about failure modes and learn from failures?*

A *How to get people to be reflective about safety, to develop mindfulness, is at the crux of the concept of patient safety and a Total Safety Culture.*

For me there was some pure luck involved. While studying at Drexel University in chemical engineering, I went to work at a DuPont Company paint plant in Philadelphia for a year and a half on the student co-op program. My safety indoctrination came from DuPont, an organization obsessed with worker safety since its earliest days as a manufacturer of gunpowder.

You were reminded about safety constantly at DuPont. Every morning I drove in past a billboard with the number of days since the last lost-time injury had occurred. It was many hundred days. Every Monday morning we had a safety talk, and once a month managers gave presentations on a safety topic. To this day, I can't walk past an open file drawer without closing it.

I'm a living, breathing example of someone who early in his career was indoctrinated into this kind of obsessive culture. Still, it took me many years to become introspective about safety.

Fortune and misfortune, life and work experiences, and personality factors all may lead people to being continuous learners and self-reflective, being watchers of their behaviors, working hard to change themselves as they recognize their weaknesses.

8 Honest self-appraisals are rare
We tend to exaggerate our abilities

Our brains don't come equipped with the "black box" recorders that preserve cockpit dialog in an airplane, but we do possess a type of "governor" to regulate our thinking — cognitive psychologists call it metacognition, metamemory, metacomprehension, or self-monitoring skills.[22] It's the ability to assess your own thinking, how well you're performing, and knowing when your judgments are likely to be accurate or in error. It's like playing devil's advocate with yourself. In healthcare "it's an incredible challenge" to maintain this sort of honest self-appraisal, says Dr. Graber.

What's true in medicine is true for the rest of us. We all contend with competing past-, present- and future-oriented thoughts that pull our attention in many different directions at once. It's hard to "regulate" them all and adhere to Thomas Jefferson's adage: "He who knows best, knows how little he knows."

Quite to the contrary, research shows we seem inclined to inflate our self-appraisals and exaggerate our performance abilities. High school students tend to see themselves as having more leadership ability, better relationship skills, and superior written communication skills than their peers. Business managers think they are more competent than the typical manager. And football players think they possess more "football savvy" than competitors on the field.[23]

It's this kind of thinking that leads to the "Peter Principle" in business, where managers are promoted to a level above their competency, and to athletes "trying to carry the team on their back" in sports. In medicine, the consequences of complacency pose an incredibly difficult challenge to patient safety, says Dr. Graber.

Complacency can allow for mental shortcuts and produce an error. But an "air of confidence" is the oxygen needed for professional decisiveness and quick-thinking — characteristics patients want to see and the public has come to expect.

"It would be deadly for us… to give up our belief in human perfectibility," writes Dr. Atul Gawande in *Complications*.[24] He knows "all doctors make terrible mistakes," yet "each time I go into a gallbladder operation I believe that with enough will and effort I can beat the odds. This isn't just professional vanity. It's a necessary part of good medicine."[25]

Medical school and residency shapes doctors' thinking that they can beat the odds. "We are taught…if you do your lessons, know your stuff, keep up, and are careful, you won't make mistakes," Dr. Lucian Leape explains. He adds, "It is hard to persuade people that this isn't enough, that there is much more to safety than just being careful."[26]

Expert Q&A *Parking bad outcomes*

A practicing general internist, the medical director of a 14-physician primary care medical group, describes "parking" bad events — another barrier to the kind of thinking that prevents error and increases patient care.[27]

Q *Do you agree with physicians who say safety is something they have built into their practice, that everything they do and think about is designed to minimize the risk of treatment — thus making patient-safety interventions redundant?*

A *Those statements usually reflect a belief that the individual physician's concern for safety is sufficient. In fact the systems we work in are so complex only a systems approach to issues of safety, and the reliability of the care delivered, can have an effect.*

For any one physician working in his/her little sphere, medical errors may seem infrequent. But we have an ability to compartmentalize bad events and park them someplace out of our everyday consciousness. It's something you learn about from experience during medical training, and in part this affects what specialties people choose to pursue.

If you work in an oversight capacity in a hospital and review all the mistakes/errors that occur, you get a different consciousness. There is growing awareness/acceptance the healthcare system greatly underperforms in the area of safety, and there are concrete things we can do to improve.

9 How to increase mindfulness

Focus on achieving small wins for patient safety

What were they thinking?

A woman learned by phone her husband had died at a local hospital. His death had been expected and the funeral had been preplanned and prepaid. The next day she took clothing and other materials needed to prepare her husband's body for viewing to the funeral home. When her family returned to the funeral home to view the body after it had been prepared, they were shocked to discover the body in the casket was not their husband and father.

The funeral director argued with the family about the identity of the person in the casket. He insisted the paperwork indicated it was their husband and father. Based on the documentation, the funeral home made a leg ID indicating it was this individual, which was pointed out to his widow. When she and the funeral director checked the body further and looked at the opposite foot, they found a tag with another man's name.

Further investigation revealed the woman's husband had been released by the hospital to the wrong funeral home and his body cremated under the other patient's identity.[28]

How can we shift from this sort of mindless thinking to more mindfulness in ourselves and others? This kind of mindful thinking is exemplified by the hypothetical case presented by Dr. Robert Wachter:

A young ward clerk took a call from the OR to send up a patient, but she couldn't find consent in the chart. The clerk wanted to be 100 percent sure the OR was calling for the right patient. She knew it would take several phone calls, and might delay the start of the case by ten minutes. She also knew the patient's surgeon, a highly respected and prominent surgeon, had something of a temper. And she saw the day's OR schedule was jammed. She decided to go ahead and make the calls to confirm everything was in order. It turned out to be just a paperwork snafu and the patient really was scheduled for surgery. Ten minutes later, she released the patient to the transporter.[29]

One of Dr. Ellen Langer's key recommendations[30] for making people more mindful is this: get them to pay more attention to how they are trying to accomplish something (such as a patient-safety goal), as opposed to focusing only on the outcome of that process (the patient-safety record).

There are many examples of how we take a process for granted and direct our focus to the outcome. Dr. Langer reminds us that starting in kindergarten the focus of schooling is on the final result. Students in Dr. Geller's university classes seem obsessed with their grades and seemingly lose sight of the important purpose of their "higher" education. Rather than focusing on the critical-thinking and problem-solving processes related to a particular theory or research finding, students memorize the facts and formulae needed to perform well on an exam.

Likewise, travel is often seen as only a means to an end. The journey can be viewed as unimportant, just as long as the destination is reached.

You can readily see the fallacy in this logic. How you complete a journey can determine whether you reach the destination in one piece. Again, the focus is on how you do it. Orient your people to the process — the steps needed to ensure patient safety every day. Emphasize their involvement in deriving corrective action plans from ongoing audits, suggestions, and incident reports.

When you see how these successive steps or "small wins" lead to an outcome such as a reduced infection rate, your sense of mindful control is enhanced. You see the outcome as hard-won through your (and others') control of the process. And by continuing to improve people's mindful attention to the process, patient injuries can be reduced even more.

So keep tracking outcomes, of course, but facilitate and support discussions of the ongoing processes needed to prevent injuries. Conversations about safety processes keep people mindful of what they must continue doing in order to keep themselves and others safe.

Expert Q&A *Use checklists judiciously*

David W. Bates, M.D. is chief of the Division of General Medicine at Brigham and Women's Hospital in Boston, Massachusetts, and professor of medicine at Harvard Medical School.

Q *You've estimated that an average internist makes several hundred decisions each day seeing patients from 8:00 a.m. to 5:00 p.m. Are cognitive errors simply inevitable given the volume and pace of daily decision-making?*

A *It is hard for us to slow down decision-making. One solution is to take some of the easy decisions out of the realm of clinicians. If a patient needs a routine mammogram and the patient is amenable, let a nurse arrange it. The physician might then be able to do something more cognitively challenging, such as caring for a patient who is short of breath.*

We do put physicians in a double bind. Pay relates to the number of visits handled. So financial incentives very clearly are in the other direction, away from slowing down.

Checklists can serve as cognitive aids, but a checklist can make things worse. Airlines noted years ago wing flaps could be in the wrong position on take-off, something a pilot could catch by looking out the window. But when the pilot's preflight checklist increased from 15 to 40 items, pilots didn't have time to look out the window: they were too busy going through the checklist. Suddenly there was a rash of crashes due to attempted take-offs with the flaps in the wrong position, which actually related to the longer checklist!

Checklists can be very helpful, but they need to be used very judiciously, especially in high-intensity medical activities. What's helpful is something like bundling. With ventilator-associated pneumonia bundling, you have four to six things to do all the time. That's manageable and not a distraction.

As part of its "100,000 Lives" campaign, the Institute for Healthcare Improvement (IHI) bundled four interventions that, combined, could reduce ventilator-associated pneumonia (VAP) — one of six target areas to reduce inpatient morbidity and mortality. The IHI VAP-prevention bundle includes the following strategies:

• Semirecumbent patient positioning to at least 30 degrees
• Ventilator weaning via periodic sedation vacations and daily assessment of extubation readiness
• Peptic ulcer disease (PUD) prophylaxis
• Deep-vein thrombosis (DVT) prophylaxis
Making sure all these things happen for an eligible patient has had a major impact.

10 Barriers to clear thinking
Pride and shame: powerful inhibitors

The fact is, in all these cases it's impossible to know precisely what the caregivers were thinking. There is no "black box" inside their heads to record self-talk and decision-making process. And a root-cause analysis would quickly run up against the complex vagaries of decision-making.

Our thoughts are indeed private, beyond the reach of a typical root-cause analysis, indeed sometimes beyond our own understanding.

"I should have immediately called Dr. Ball for backup," writes Dr. Atul Gawande, recounting a botched emergency tracheotomy in *Complications*. "But for whatever reasons — hubris, inattention, wishful thinking, hesitation, or the uncertainty of the moment — I let the opportunity pass."[31]

Thus, medicine is left with few lessons learned from decision-making errors that result from faulty thinking. That's unless people are willing to let you come "inside" so to speak, and talk about their personal thought processes. Usually that door remains shut — off limits. "Physicians are uncomfortable discussing diagnostic error," says Dr. Mark Graber.[32] When it comes to making errors and mistakes, pride and shame are powerful inhibitors.

Malpractice suits are another major barrier to learning. In the Veterans Health Administration, tort claims related to diagnostic errors were twice as common as claims related to medication errors.[33] By using these errors to attack doctors, doctors retreat from acknowledging and discussing them publicly.

So in the broad realm of patient-safety issues, scant attention goes to cognitive failures — despite diagnostic errors of decision-making being a major issue. For example, in the Harvard Medical Practice Study, diagnostic errors were the second-leading cause of adverse events.[34]

Out of sight, out of mind. "We have an ability to compartmentalize bad events and park them someplace out of our everyday consciousness," says one physician.[35] That seems to be especially true when the error or bad event draws into question one's own decision-making. Nothing is more personal than one's own thoughts. And nothing is more relevant to professional competency in healthcare than critical thinking skills.

Other factors — activators and consequences as described in Chapter 2 — influence thinking and impact a patient's safety. Take

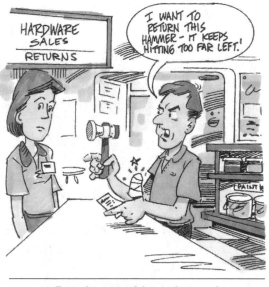

People pass blame beyond themselves.

the nurse who strode into the patient's room ready to give him his dose of clonazepam, only to discover she had the wrong patient.

It turns out, due to a bed shortage, patient Mr. J was to be moved down the hall, and Mr. X, a seizure patient scheduled to be transferred out of the neuro-ICU that afternoon, was to move into that room. The room change was made on the hospital's computer before the moves were actually executed. But the computer showed the nurse Mr. X was in that room and due for his clonazepam.

The most obvious error (and most immediate activator of the nurse's actions) was the patient's relocation was recorded in the computer system before it actually happened. But the nurse failed to correctly identify the patient when she began to administer the medication. When first entering the room, she didn't ask for his name, nor examine his wristband in search of the two unique identifiers.

Brushing aside questions of patient identity could be a case of caregiver unease with uncertainty. What patient wants a nurse or physician standing bedside, hemming and hawing, "Do I have this right? I don't know, what do you think?"

Patients who are vulnerable through injury or disease take comfort in displays of confidence and authority by their caregivers. Some might even be said to feed off it. Most expect it, and passively if not overtly press for it. The result is what Dr. Graber calls a "cognitive disposition to respond."[36] Or as he told us in an interview, a disposition to fish around, find it, fix it, and move on.

The nurse who almost gave the wrong patient the wrong medicine very well could have been pressed for time, responsible for too many beds, and/or drained at the end of a long shift. Production pressures, patient ratios, and fatigue all affect how caregivers think on the job.

Production pressures in healthcare keep ratcheting up. It's indeed a challenge to maintain mental alertness in the face of pressure to run hospitals at 100-percent capacity, with every bed filled with the sickest possible patients who are discharged at the first sign they are stable, or the pressure to leave no operating room unused and to keep moving through the schedule for each room as fast as possible.[37]

So we have a hyped-up climate in healthcare: abbreviated office visits, impatient listening, frayed nerves and hurried decision-making. Psychologists call it premature closure. "There's pressure to move on," says Dr. Graber. "Pressure from the patient for a definitive, confident answer. Pressure to solve each problem quickly and be done with it. It takes time to reexamine your thinking and reexamine the facts. It also motivation, and can drive people crazy."

Heavy workloads, a corollary to production pressures, exact a toll on clear-headed thinking — and on patient safety. Recent research shows in a given unit the optimal workload for a nurse was four patients. Increasing the workload to six resulted in patients being 14 percent more likely to die within 30 days of admission. A workload of eight patients versus four was associated with a 31-percent increase in mortality.[38]

Production pressure also contributes to extended work hours and fatigue. Most nurses no longer work traditional eight-hour days, evening or night shifts. Over one-third of the shifts studied in one research survey were scheduled for 12.5 hours or longer, and 43 percent of the shifts exceeded 12.5 consecutive hours. Nurses in this study rarely left work at the end of their scheduled shift, and they averaged almost an extra hour per day.[39]

What mental toll results? Such things as forgetfulness, slowed reaction time, reduced vigilance, poor communication, apathy, impulsive decision-making. Tasks may be begun well but performance deteriorates with increasing rapidity. Persistent attempts at ineffective solutions occur. Loss of situational awareness occurs, where activities mistakenly judged to be nonessential are neglected. Involuntary microsleeps occur. And cognitive deficits may be masked by stimulation — caffeine, etc.[40]

Healthcare worker fatigue poses a significant threat to patient safety, according to background provided for JCAHO's draft candidate 2007 National Patient Safety Goal 19 — prevent patient harm associated with healthcare worker fatigue (for hospitals and critical access hospital programs). Fatigue diminishes staff's capacity to recognize important but subtle changes in a patient's condition, according to JCAHO. To meet this patient-safety goal, organizations are expected to manage work hours and periods of on-call to minimize fatigue, and staff schedules reflect known affects of sleep physiology. Plus, the organization supports a work ethic that considers fatigue as an unacceptable risk to patient care.[41]

Expert Q&A *"A lot of physicians think they can handle fatigue..."*

David W. Bates, M.D., is chief of the Division of General Medicine at Brigham and Women's Hospital in Boston, Mass., and professor of medicine at Harvard Medical School.

Q *You've studied physician fatigue and found that housestaff officers made 30 percent more serious errors when they were fatigued than when they were not. What can a patient-safety officer in a hospital do about physician fatigue? Doesn't it just come with the territory?*

A *No, it doesn't come with the territory. Patient-safety personnel and hospital and clinical leadership can stand up for rules and policies about length of shifts. Extended-duty shifts, those greater than 24 hours, are a key issue. Limiting the hours worked per week is useful but doesn't fully address the length of shifts.*

Performance deteriorates after a night of missed sleep. The thing to do is not allow physicians to stay up all night. We did an intervention in the ICU where internists got regular sleep and the program was quite effective.

A lot of physicians think they can handle fatigue, but in fact everyone's performance declines, and most people are not aware of how their performance declines. There is a pretty substantial fall-off in performance after sleep deprivation; after being up all night it's like being intoxicated. But physicians will say, "I'm aware, I'm taking extra care." The increase in errors doesn't bear that out.

Hidden pressures

Long shifts, long work weeks and too few nurses for too many patients are some of the more overt contributors to faulty, fuzzy thinking. There are also more hidden influences. Take the fourth-year medical student who observed a catheter being inserted into a patient prior to surgery; he was surprised to see no efforts were made to perform "sterile prep" prior to insertion, but decided not to mention it to anyone in the OR.

What was he thinking?

He might have been responding to some of medicine's implicit rules, customs and rituals. There is enormous respect for hierarchy, and reluctance to raise an alarm when one merely suspects, but is not sure, that something is amiss. There's a tendency to let it slide and say, "Oh, it's probably OK."[42] In this case, the student was new to the setting and didn't know if different practices were used in pediatric patients. But he did know his place as low man on the totem pole.

11 Training improves self-monitoring skills
But techniques can encourage mindfulness or mindlessness

Researchers at Cornell University conducted studies in the late 1990s that demonstrated training — in the form of techniques for testing the veracity of deductive reasoning — can provide individuals with improved metacognitive skills to assess their own performance more correctly.[43]

There's more than technique involved, too. Did you ever think about how your style as a trainer or coach for patient safety can encourage either mindlessness or mindfulness? Dr. Ellen Langer made this case: When facts are presented unconditionally as an absolute truth, alternative ways of thinking about something are stifled.[44] She backed this up with an interesting study. A collection of objects was introduced in an ordinary, unconditional way to one group, as for example, "This is a dog's chew toy." For the second group, objects were introduced conditionally with the extra phrase "could be," as in, "This could be a dog's chew toy."

After the objects were introduced, the groups were asked to complete some survey forms. Then the experimenter announced the survey could not continue because the wrong instructions had been given and no spare forms were available. At that point several subjects suggested the rubber chew toy could be used as an eraser to correct the flawed forms. Interestingly, this resourceful idea came only from the conditional group — those told, "This could be a dog's chew toy."

Do you discuss patient-safety rules as unconditional mandates? Or do you focus on safety principles that imply certain guidelines but can be customized?

It's obvious which approach stimulates more creativity and ownership among individuals and work teams. The uncertainty of the second approach allows people to use their minds in figuring out how to adapt a safety principle for a particular situation. In turn, they feel like they own the solution they came up with, and they will be committed to mindfully follow the personalized procedures.

Regulatory robots

We asked Lori Ann Paine, RN, the patient-safety coordinator for The Johns Hopkins Hospital, how she felt about using accreditation requirements to motivate compliance to patient-safety initiatives. She was to the point:

"You get people slipping into a glazed, half-asleep robot mode. 'OK, we've got to do it.' Regulatory requirements create an external locus of control. You don't get a feeling of ownership.

"We're trying to change our culture (at The Johns Hopkins

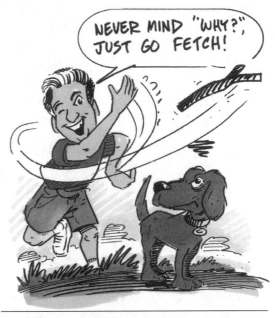

Without education, training can feel degrading.

Hospital), to create a just environment where there is a safe feeling that you can report errors. Regulatory requirements feel far more punitive. You don't want to tell staff this is the reason you're doing patient safety."

Remember, the problem with direct persuasion, such as rule compliance, is it comes across as someone else's idea. And it can give the impression the desired behavior is primarily for someone else's benefit.

Training can't always "fix" thinking

Too often "retraining" or "discipline" is selected impulsively to correct a discrepancy between what people do and what we want them to do. Perhaps they don't know what's expected, or they don't have the right resources or enough time. Sometimes people are rewarded for the wrong behavior, or ignored or punished for performing the safe way. Useful feedback may be missing.

In these cases, people know what to do, but they just aren't doing it. They are "consciously incompetent." The problem is not lack of knowledge or skill. Training is not the answer. You need to analyze and change organizational systems, workplace conditions, and interpersonal relations.

In their practical performance-improvement book, Robert Mager and Peter Pipe suggest a number of ways to get the performance you want before concluding that formal training is needed.[45] Ask yourself these three questions:

1) Can the task be simplified?

Before developing a training program to improve patient safety, make sure all possible engineering "fixes" have been implemented. Explore the many ways the environment could be changed to reduce physical effort, reach, and repetition. Entertain ways to make the job more user-friendly before deciding what behaviors are needed to prevent injury.

2) Is there a skill discrepancy?

What about those times when staff members are "unconsciously incompetent" — they really don't know how to work safely? This might call for training. But Mager and Pipe claim most behavioral discrepancies are not caused by a genuine lack of skill. Usually, people can work safely if conditions and consequences are right. So training should really be the least-used approach for corrective action.

3) What kind of training is needed?

If you determine that someone has forgotten how to perform a task, a skill maintenance program may be in order. This is the rationale behind periodic emergency training. Fortunately, emergencies don't happen very often, but since they don't, people need to go through the motions just to "stay in practice."

Skill maintenance training is also needed when a person gets plenty of practice doing the wrong thing. Here, practice only reinforces a bad (or risky) habit. For example, most people know how to drive a vehicle safely, and once showed little at-risk driving. But safe driving often deteriorates over time.

Behavior-based feedback is critical for solving both of these skill discrepancies, especially when desired skills have deteriorated into poor habits (as in the driving example). A behavior-based coach is needed. The coach needs to systematically complete a critical behavior checklist while watching for safe

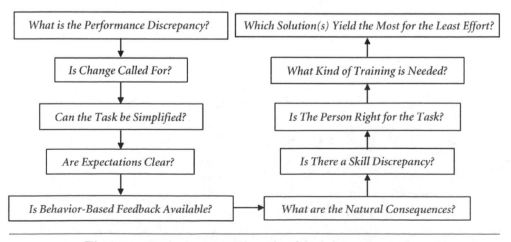

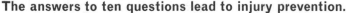

The answers to ten questions lead to injury prevention.

versus at-risk actions, and then give both supportive and corrective feedback.

Of course, there is also the training needed to introduce a new procedure or process.

Remember, if you're not getting the performance you want from employees, the reasons will often be found in the work environment or in the task itself. Don't impulsively assume the answer lies in training or discipline. Analyze the situation, the behavior, and the individuals involved to prioritize possible solutions.

12   How to facilitate a "success seeking" mindset

Building a robust mindset for patient safety

During my (ESG) 40 years of university teaching, I've noticed some students possess a "need to achieve," while others portray a "need to avoid failure."

Failure avoiders study only minimally to avoid failure, and are not "happy campers." Those who "work to achieve" enjoy my class much more. They view it as an opportunity to earn a good grade, even an opportunity to learn.

This dichotomy of working to achieve versus working to avoid failure is based on classic research conducted in the 1950s and 1960s by Richard Atkinson and David McClelland.[46] Atkinson's original theory identified four types of individuals: success seekers, overstrivers, failure avoiders, and failure accepters. All four exhibit personality states that influence the self-talk we've discussed in this chapter and the outcome of your patient-safety efforts.

Think about these personality types in the make-up of your patient-safety team: Success seekers are the most desirable participants. These individuals show the highest levels of self-efficacy, personal control, and optimism. With the high expectancy for success and low fear of failure, success seekers respond to setbacks with optimistic persistence, self-assurance, and a sense of personal control.

It's generally better to be an overstriver than a failure avoider or failure accepter, but the high fear of failure among overstrivers leads to self-doubt. These individuals experience high levels of distress, low perceptions of personal control, and unstable self-esteem.

As you can imagine, failure avoiders have low expectations for success and thus avoid challenges. They are unsure of themselves, and are overly anxious and pessimistic about the future. Failure accepters are actually better adjusted than failure avoiders. Their acceptance leads generally to apathy, not anxiety. But from your team perspective, failure accepters are least desirable — they have simply given up.

So how would you classify yourself in terms of these four person states? How would you categorize your team members? Would you place some people in one category with regard to patient safety, but in another category when it comes to other professional responsibilities? Have you seen people, perhaps yourself, change from one state to another as the result of certain experiences? Keep in mind that environmental conditions, work contexts, and cultures determine the number of safety success seekers in an organization.

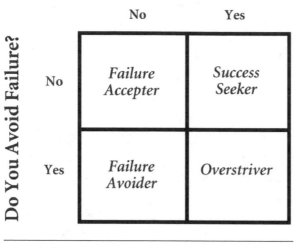

Do You Seek Success?

	No	Yes
No	*Failure Accepter*	*Success Seeker*
Yes	*Failure Avoider*	*Overstriver*

(left axis: **Do You Avoid Failure?**)

Thinking success or failure affects attitude and behavior.

It's obvious we need to find ways to facilitate a success-seeking mindset — both in individuals and teams. The more safety success seekers in your organization, the greater the probability of achieving and maintaining a high level of patient care, and low level of error. Let's consider ways to increase the number of safety success seekers on a team, in a unit, or throughout an organization.

Traditional safety programs in general industry emphasize failure avoidance over positive achievements. They all share these attributes:

• Key indices of safe performance focus on avoiding failure (from numbering injuries to work-compensation costs).

• Safety rewards or financial bonuses based on days without an injury or incident make failure avoidance a primary motivator. In healthcare, a parallel target would be days in a unit without a hospital-acquired infection.

• Organizational rankings in terms of safety are based on who has the lowest number of incidents, and a reactive failure-avoidance stance takes precedence over success seeking.

• Management considers "incident investigation" the key job responsibility of the company safety pro, giving priority status to avoiding failure.

• Managers summarize safety performance with statistics and numbers centering around losses and failures, thus putting clear and obvious emphasis on failure avoidance.

The obvious antidote is to focus on safety achievement rather than injury avoidance. Easier said than done, we admit. The only way to put an achievement spin on safety is to define proactive things to do for patient safety, and then hold people accountable for achieving them. An achievement-based accountability system should put more focus on positive consequences for accomplishment, from interpersonal recognition to group celebrations. Plus, your safety scoring system should be based on leading indicators — activities accomplished to prevent injury.[47]

Imagine the alternatives

Imagine a patient-safety meeting that begins with a presentation of various process accomplishments for prevent harm. You might discuss:
- The number of environmental hazards removed
- Close-call reports reviewed
- Safety audits completed
- Interpersonal coaching sessions conducted
- Safety suggestions received and implemented, and
- Percentage of safe behaviors observed per work team.

Moreover, imagine the meeting facilitator asking participants to state publicly what they have done for patient safety since the last meeting. Imagine patient-safety teams recognized for what they do to prevent harm and reduce risks. And imagine the safety portion of a performance appraisal including a checklist of safety accomplishments.

With these transitions, it's not difficult to imagine cultivating achievement-oriented thinking about patient safety — and thereby increasing the number of "safety success seekers."

13 Mindsets make or break "investigations"
Are you fact-finding or fault-finding?

First off, stop using that word "investigation." Doesn't this imply a hunt for some single cause or person to blame for a particular error event or failure, as in "criminal investigation"?

How can we promote fact-finding over fault-finding with a term like "investigation" defining our job assignment?

To truly learn more about how to prevent risks and reduce errors from an analysis of a patient-safety incident, we need to approach the task with a different mindset. Don't call it an "investigation." It's an "incident analysis." This simple substitution of words can have substantial impact. We can get more staff participation and in fact, reap more benefits from the entire process. Here are five reasons to change our thinking, and our language:

1 – Gain a broader understanding

A common myth in the safety field holds that harm is caused by one critical factor — the root cause. "Ask enough questions and you'll arrive at the critical factor behind an injury." Some claim you ask "Why?" five times to find the root cause. Do you really believe there is a single root cause?

Consider the three sides of "The Safety Triad": environment, behavior and person factors that affect patient safety. Environment factors include tools, equipment, engineering design, climate and housekeeping. Then you have the behaviors, the actions of everyone relating to an incident. Finally, there are the personal, internal states of the people involved — their attitudes, perceptions, and personality characteristics.

Take a systems approach in your analysis of environment, behavior and person factors. Then decide which of these factors can be changed to reduce the chance of another unfortunate incident. Environment factors are usually easiest to define and improve, followed by behavior factors. Most difficult to define and change directly are the person factors, but many of these internal feelings can be affected positively by properly influencing behaviors.

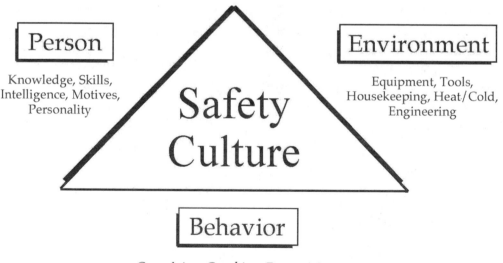

Person	Environment
Knowledge, Skills, Intelligence, Motives, Personality	Equipment, Tools, Housekeeping, Heat/Cold, Engineering

Safety Culture

Behavior

Complying, Coaching, Recognizing, Communicating, Demonstrating "Actively Caring"

Environment, behavior, and person factors all affect safety.

---

2 – Improve communication

To find and correct the potential contributors to an incident, people need to think about the various environmental, behavioral and personal factors and then talk openly about them. But this won't happen when people are thinking "investigation" — to find a single reason for the "failure." People want nothing to do with failure.

It's human nature. Kids will blame the other kid — "He made me do it."

Adults will just keep their mouths shut. To get people to open up, we need to approach incident analysis as an opportunity for success. Let's get away from the perspective of incident-equals-failure. The mindset should be how an incident gives us the chance to learn and improve. This can lead to more reports of personal close calls where patients were almost harmed. The more we report and analyze, the more opportunity we have to correct problems before harm actually reaches a patient.

3 – Increase involvement

You can expect more participation in incident reporting and analysis if you involve staff in thinking about the actual correction phase of the process. People will contribute more if their ideas are considered in the outcome. Of course, administrators need to approve and support the corrections recommended by those on the frontlines. But staff on the floor know more than anyone else about what it will take to make environmental, behavioral and personal factors more safe. Use their critical thinking skills and you'll motivate more ownership and involvement in the entire process.

4 – Apply systems solutions

Here's how an "investigation" is usually wrapped up: The patient-safety manager or equivalent person in the hierarchy presents a report to management, and the recommended solution to eliminating the "root cause" is implemented in the unit where the incident occurred. Equipment might be replaced, or a certain employee might be "retrained" or even punished (incorrectly considered "discipline" in the safety literature).

You'll get broader thinking and involvement in an incident analysis process if corrective action plans are applied across all the "microsystems" that make up an organization. This also promotes systems thinking over the piecemeal, "band-aid" perspective common to so many organizational cultures. Think about the bigger picture. Use the results of an incident analysis to improve relevant environmental, behavioral and personal factors hospital-wide, when feasible. This sends the kind of actively caring message that not only promotes the right kind of constructive thinking, but also increases participation.

5 – Promote accountability

Both the quantity and quality of constructive thinking in incident analysis depend on the outcome numbers used to evaluate success or failure. Remember, most bottom-line measures don't give you nearly enough information about why numbers are rising or falling.

Instead, keep track of the various components of incident analysis. Monitor the number of close calls and patient-safety incidents reported. Track the number of corrective actions implemented for environmental, behavioral and personal factors. Now you have an accountability system that facilitates constructive thinking and participation.

Keep your mindset on successfully completing these various steps of the process. Keep score of your process achievements rather than only waiting to see final output numbers rise or fall — infection rates, medication errors, patient-safety perception survey results. Instead of waiting to see what comes out of your patient-safety pipeline, you need to track the activities occurring along the way. Safety professionals call these proactive measures "leading indicators."

Analyze close calls

When you analyze a sentinel event, or whatever definition you use for an adverse event, you are reacting to a crisis. This reactive behavior is at times a type of regulatory requirement, or a matter of internal policy. When you consider close calls or "near hits," however, you can prevent harm before it occurs.

This proactive thinking unfortunately does not have many natural incentives. Indeed, it seems most natural to avoid thinking about our near hits and hide them from others. After all, a close call usually reflects thoughtless or careless behavior, and most people don't want to admit being thoughtless, careless, or unsafe — unless they have to (such as after harm actually reaches the patient).

Where is the support for proactive thinking? Policies and procedures should be implemented to motivate continual proactive patient-safety behavior. For example, staff need to communicate their "close calls" to others and develop corrective actions before similar incidents result in patient harm. Proactive thinking and corrective action should address the three basic factors contributing to near hits and patient harm — the environmental, behavioral and personal factors mentioned above.

FAQ *How do you respond to the thinking that errors are inevitable, system vulnerabilities are inevitable, healthcare systems are just too complex and unpredictable. So why bother with serious investments in time and money for patient safety?*

A mindset of inevitability is tantamount to learned helplessness or failure acceptance. This mindset is clearly detrimental to patient safety and causes distress. We experience stress (beneficial motivation) when we are in control, but experience distress (debilitating motivation) when the perception of control is lacking. Thus, it's essential to focus on things that can be done to improve patient safety. This relates of course to the notion of seeking success rather than avoiding failure.

The mindset that accidents are inevitable is detrimental to patient safety. First, we recommend using the term accident only when knowledge is not available for preventing the injury. In more cases than not, we knew enough to prevent the mishap. We just did not execute appropriately, or take the necessary precautions.

The prevention of errors is complex because the system is complex. It is dynamic and intricate at the same time. Environmental, behavioral and personal factors contribute to errors, and we need to identify these if we want to reduce errors. Can this be a challenge? Yes, but it can be done through a proactive mindset, and open and frank communication leading to intervention development and interdependent thinking.

FAQ How do you move mindsets from worry and anxiety over safety to personal control and optimism?

This question addresses the critical distinction between avoiding failure and seeking success. This is a motivational question. In other words, people perform to achieve positive consequences or avoid negative consequences. Soon and certain consequences are most motivational, whether they are positive or negative. So why do we want positive consequences or a success-seeking mindset? Because people feel better (free and in control) when working for positive consequences than when working to achieve negative consequences.

But this does not mean worry about potential negative consequences is bad. Such worrisome thinking should motivate proactive behavior. When people are concerned about negative consequences, we have them thinking about ways to avoid those negative consequences. We do this by implementing proactive or prevention intervention. And we increase the acceptance of these interventions by discussing them in terms of seeking success.

In other words, we need to think and talk about what we do for patient safety. Sure, we want to avoid negative consequences, but to do that we need to think and act proactively. And we need to think and communicate in terms of achievement rather than avoiding failure. It's all about putting people in control in ways that enable them to believe they are in control. This requires a success-seeking mindset, which is enabled through communication and intervention that focuses on activities that prevent the negative consequences that cause worry.

CHAPTER 5 *Seeing*

In this chapter you'll learn:

1 The risk of premature cognitive commitment

The hazards we miss when our minds are made up

What we have in the cases described in the following list of bullets are, yes, "failures to communicate," but more specifically breakdowns psychologists refer to as "premature cognitive commitment."[1] Call it tunnel vision, or cognitive short-cutting. Whatever — these kinds of automatic responses to biased perceptions of evidence can and do put patients at risk.

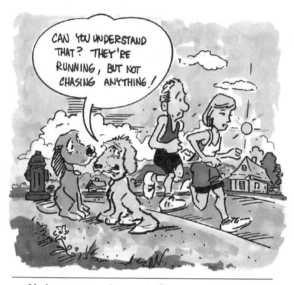

Unique experience influences unique interpretation, and vice versa.

• The nurse and pharmacist who blindly gave a blind man instructions on how to self-inject (Described in Chapter 4)? Their "premature" assessment perhaps came from an unthinking assumption: they were simply discharging another patient.[2]

• The nurse who attempted to give Mr. J the medication intended for Mr. X (Chapter 4)? Her premature commitment to administer the clonazepam was based on erroneous information she received from a computer log. The monitor indicated the room was occupied by Mr. X, with Mr. J having moved to another room, although the transfer hadn't occurred yet. Apparently the computer chart was all the evidence the nurse needed to make a "commitment" to the identity of the patient; she never actually asked the man his name before proceeding.[3]

• A clinician misinterpreted a patient's wristband color, it is believed, because the caregiver involved worked in facilities in which yellow-colored wristbands had different meanings. This led to a premature commitment to yellow as possessing a certain meaning.[4]

• An intern ignored repeated suggestions from a pharmacist that he had misread a steroids prescription. Perhaps he clung to a premature conclusion associated with the "hidden curriculum"[5] in medical education. Implicit rules that devalue input from non-physician professionals and discourage asking for assistance, even after it's been recommended.[6]

In all these cases, caregivers were "seeing" what they expected to see. So sure of their assessment, so committed to it, they didn't realize they were acting prematurely — and putting patients at risk.

"The risks we see in healthcare are the risks we're prepared for," says Martin J. Hatlie, president of the Partnership for Patient Safety. The nurse and the pharmacist were not prepared to encounter a blind man at discharge. The nurse was expecting a computerized recordkeeping error. The clinician was not ready for a yellow wristband with a meaning different from his past experience. The intern was of no mind to question his own judgment.

It's not humanly possible to see the curves coming our way every day, all the more so in healthcare, where every patient brings a unique set of risks. But we can do a better job of seeing what's going on around us. We can take more active control over our perceptions — just as we can control our thinking — to allow us to better identify and make necessary adjustments to risk.

Recognizing premature cognitive commitment is a good place to start, because it can have a damaging effect on your patient-safety efforts in a number of ways.

1) Since it's premature — occurring before adequate data collection, analysis and verification — it blocks constructive learning. For example, it's difficult to teach patient-safety principles and methods to people possessing these preconceived perceptions:

• All patient-safety answers lie with management and its systems.

• Anything to do with the human side of patient safety is warm and fuzzy experimentation.

• Patient safety is simply another accreditation requirement or a passing fad.

2) Being cognitive — a biased mental processing — can lead to especially detrimental global stereotypes. As in:

• Patient-safety officers are reminiscent of other middle manager types; well-meaning but without authority.

• Patient-safety teams are like many work groups; hastily-constructed and rudderless.

• Patient-safety meetings are, well, like most meetings — a chance to catch up on microsleep.

3) Finally, we are talking about a commitment — a relatively fixed way of looking at things that filters the information we receive, and shapes how we act. This leads to the third effect: When we adopt narrow and premature definitions and concepts we limit choice and personal control. When we become committed to a single-minded perception (patient safety is a passing fad, a quick fix for accreditation compliance), we are not open to information that runs counter to it. (Think of the intern's reaction to the pharmacist's recommendations.) We are not apt to participate in interventions when asked. Why should we, when we believe we have no real control over an intervention's success or failure?

In other words, we commit ourselves to an initial impression without the

Expert Q&A *Working with blinders on*

A nurse epidemiologist who completed a year-long executive fellowship in patient safety describes several perceptual traps.

Q *What are typical examples of working with blinders on — erroneous assumptions, complacency, over-confidence?*

A *For starters we should set the proper tone and admit — without blaming or scolding — the many errors made that do patients harm. In healthcare we get it, we screw up, we know it. But no one I know ever goes to work saying, "I think I'll kill a patient today." Individuals make mistakes because the system sets them up for failure even when they are acting safely.*

That said, here's an erroneous assumption in healthcare: believing many, if not all, of our patients are literate and will understand our written

benefit of mindful seeing, and that distorts how we process and respond to subsequent information. We misread the prescription. Misinterpret the wristband. Misidentify patients. Talk right past patients, as though we don't see them.

We hope you see the problems large and small created by premature cognitive commitment. At the level of individual interactions, these faulty perceptions increase risks to patients and cause preventable harm. On a global scale, this kind of narrow-sightedness can scuttle an organization's attempt to build a Patient-Safety Culture.

Here's another development you need to "see": Patient care and safety are improving as technologies such as medication bar coding and computerized physician order entry systems slowly gain greater acceptance. But technology can also create new blind spots for caregivers, as we show later. To summarize: A culture vigilant to matters of patient safety is not possible until a fundamental change occurs in the way caregivers see risk. This requires releasing premature conclusions and commitment. Taking the blinders off.

Caregivers are extraordinarily perceptive individuals, whether it's diagnosing chest pain, reading X-rays, studying cultures, recognizing changes in patients' conditions, or identifying patients at risk for falls or suicide. The remainder of this chapter describes how to harness the power of visual acuity to boost, not subvert, patient-safety efforts.

instructions. Due to high demands on our time, we often rely on written material to educate patients. But providing illiterate patients with a copy of their discharge instructions, or handing them a brochure explaining how to manage their diabetes or hypertension is useless when they can't read.

Complacency due to familiarity can often lead to medication errors. Even in acute settings patients may have lengthy stays. Nurses assigned to these same patients day in and day out may be tempted to skip the 5 Rs (Right medication, Right patient, Right dose, Right route, Right time) taught to us for proper medication administration.

Over-confidence can occur when caregivers forget that, they too, are human. We often ignore personal fatigue and illness because we see we perform the same even when tired or sick. Over-confidence in our abilities may lead us to take shortcuts because we're tired and opt for convenience rather than safety.

2 Selective perception: How it distorts risk assessment

There is nothing straightforward about how we see

Either we see something, or we don't, right? Wrong. Information reaches us only after being filtered through our past experiences, prejudices, as well as what we expect to see or think we will see — those premature cognitive commitments. This filtering process — called Selective Perception — leaves us with blind spots — a human fallibility particularly dangerous in healthcare where observation skills are so crucial.[7]

The following "hazard recognition traps" stem from the ways our perception is selective and subjective. Based on the following list of traps, compose a checklist of filters and biases to discuss in a group.

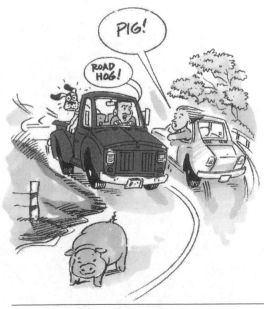

Biased perceptions can cause dangerous inattention.

Which, if any, might prevent clear and fair assessments of patient-safety incident reports, the analyses of close calls and injury events, and risk surveillance procedures.

Premature closure: Once a diagnosis is reached, clinicians have a tendency to stop thinking, says Dr. Mark Graber. This is possibly the most common cognitive error in internal medicine.[8] An existing diagnosis has what Graber calls "almost infinite inertia." A variation of premature closure is to perceive the correctness of another's diagnosis or presentation of information without re-examining the facts and independently re-thinking what is being presented to you.

Fundamental attribution error[9]: A form of "I'm OK, You're Not OK." If we see someone else err, we're likely to explain away their behavior by pointing to personal characteristics or attributes (such as personality, intelligence, status). If we find ourselves making a similar error, we're more likely to attribute it to circumstances beyond our control. It's perceptual self-protection. Watch for these misdirected perceptions in incident reporting and interviews.

Belief in a just world[10]: Many people see the world as a just and fair place, implied by the statement, "What goes around comes around." In other words, we get what we deserve. When harm seems undeserved — when a passive, vulnerable patient (especially a child) is neglected, misidentified or unnecessarily inflicted with pain — strong emotions are aroused. This sense of "injustice" accounts in part for the increased media, political and institutional attention now directed to patient safety.

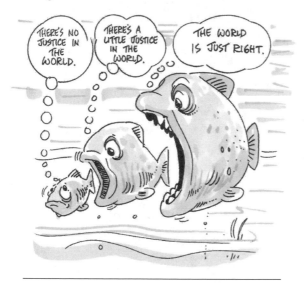

Position affects just-world perceptions.

The perception of a just world also contributes to the common belief, "It won't happen to me." Since most of us believe we are essentially good and therefore undeserving of a slip (mental lapse) or mistake (incorrect decision), we expect the "other guy" to be more apt to err. Everyday experiences usually support this perception. Errors do happen, but not to most caregivers on a daily basis, even when they take risks.

Watch for this largely unspoken observation that "People get what's coming to them" in incident investigations. The more serious the consequences of an incident, the more likely we are to judge the behavior of the individual who erred as wrong.

Acceptable consequences: The relative convenience and security of not speaking up or "stopping the line" for patient safety are easy to see. On the other hand, what are the rewards for crossing the line and confronting authorities above you? In fact, positive rewards for doing the right thing are more difficult to discern. They will likely be delayed (someone thanks you later) if they do happen, and often are invisible (the patient is not harmed — "it's like nothing happened"). We are motivated by what we see as soon, certain, and obvious consequences, and risky actions are often seen as having acceptable consequences with these characteristics.

Hindsight bias: This is Monday morning quarterbacking. After learning the outcome, people review events leading up to that outcome as though they were expected or obvious, although in real time the events perplexed those involved. Again, this bias can surface during incident analyses. Difficult decisions are more likely to be cast as errors after an undesirable outcome occurs. "Ah, but the outcome wouldn't have occurred but for the errors in judgment."

Contextual bias: The context or environmental surroundings in our visual field influence the way we are able, or unable, to see a risk. Risk perception in an emergency department is different from an operating room, different in intensive care, different in the cafeteria or parking lot. When studying a patient-safety incident or near-harm case, consider the context in which it occurred, and how environmental stimuli might have affected perceptions of risk at the time.

Framing: This bias is due to "packaging," the way information is presented to you. The way you "see it" — your opinion about a piece of information — may differ if it's delivered by a CEO you don't trust versus a chief medical officer you respect.

Anchoring error: Past events or incidents, especially recent ones, bias the way we see current events. For example, a series of preventable patient falls occur. Poor housekeeping creating tripping hazards is a common thread in these cases. The next time a patient falls, what do you think will be seen as the cause?

Choice: Risks we choose to take (driving to work each day) appear less dangerous than those hazards we feel compelled to endure (like treating a patient with HIV, TB or another infectious disease).

For example, people who feel choice over their shift assignment (they could work any shift they wanted to) would likely see less risk (and experience less stress) in working the night shift, even if it meant walking through a parking garage in the dark. Also, employees who feel more choice regarding taking on an assignment like observing patient-safety-related behaviors in a unit, or joining a patient-safety committee, typically are more motivated and feel less distressed.

Familiarity/Habituation: The more we encounter a potential risk, the less dangerous it appears to us. This desensitization process is a type of self-defense mechanism, allowing people to endure prolonged stress. But it can be a dangerous one.

You can appreciate this principle by recalling your safety-related behaviors when you first started to drive and comparing them with your current driving. As experience increases our perception of control, it also increases the possibility of risk-taking.

Familiarity is probably a more powerful determinant of how we assess risk than choice. The more information and experience we have regarding a risk, the less threatening it appears.

Recall how attentive you were to potential hazards when first introduced to high-tech equipment in your workplace. Remember also how quickly your perceived risk was lowered as operating the equipment became more familiar, and you adjusted your behavior accordingly. When driving a car, for example, most of us quickly shifted from "both hands on the wheel and no distracting radio or conversation" to "one hand on the wheel, loud radio, and ongoing verbal interaction."

Control: The risks we observe to be under our control cause much less alarm than risks that we don't understand and see as uncontrollable.[11]

Many safety education and training programs throughout general industry describe risks and give the impression they are controllable. Indeed, corporate cultures often state a vision or goal of "zero accidents," implying complete control over the factors that cause errors. And so in the process of convincing employees the causes of risk, error and injury are understood and controllable (enabling prevention of all accidents), employees see risk as less of a threat. A subtle sense of complacency can creep in over time.

③ Don't focus on one root cause
"We tend to only see slices of activity"

"Healthcare is so interdependent," says Julianne Morath, chief operating officer of the Children's Hospitals and Clinics of Minnesota. She explains how patients, instruments, supplies, medicine, records, test results all flow in a series of hand-offs between individuals, teams, units, departments, floors and facilities. "We tend to only see slices of this activity," she observes.

Analyzing adverse events presents an opportunity to "edit the slices together." So does engaging in systems thinking exercises when a group, or even individuals one-on-one, dissect patient-safety issues. Whether you're investigating an incident or analyzing a system, your powers of perception must be fog-free. Break out your checklist of perception filters and be sure they are all in the "off" position.

Look for multiple causes

"Root cause" is a longstanding concept among medical professionals, especially when conducting a root-cause analysis of sentinel events, as well as other incidents. Don't make the mistake we've often seen in general industry, where safety professionals perceive the objective of an incident analysis is to find the root cause — the single most critical factor that caused the incident. They examine the environmental context carefully and solicit opinions from everyone who might have witnessed the incident. They ask "why" an incident occurred multiple times to peel away non-issues. This process is sound. The problem arises when investigators narrowly set their sights for the root cause.

Can we convince you there is really not one root cause to uncover. Multiple errors usually align to produce the unwanted outcome. Naturally this is a more difficult phenomenon to observe.

Root-cause analyses test our observation skills. Proceed with care, with eyes wide open to all possible contributing factors. To conduct open and fair root-cause analyses, let's start by understanding how difficult it is to truly establish a cause-and-effect relationship.

What is cause and effect?

Real-world events — both desirable and undesirable — have causes. Events do not happen by themselves or for no reason. In fact, the notion that every event has a specific cause is a basic assumption of science. Researchers apply the scientific method to search for the causes of events or behaviors. But this is easier said than done. Let's review three criteria, each of which is required to make a scientifically valid connection between cause and effect.[12]

Covariation: This is the easiest criterion to establish. It means the presumed causal factor must be present when the event (or behavior) occurs.

This criterion for identifying a cause-and-effect relationship can be measured with a survey or by behavioral sampling. Surveys can show correlations between two or more factors, and observations of a behavior within specific surroundings can demonstrate that a behavior and an environmental factor covary — they occur together in time and space.

Time-order relationship: Demonstrating a cause-and-effect relationship requires more than covariation. It is also necessary to determine which variable, factor, or event occurred first. This criterion can only be satisfied when the presumed causal factor is manipulated (as an independent variable) and its impact is subsequently observed in another factor (the dependent variable).

No other explanation: Covariation and time-order relationships are necessary, but not sufficient for defining a valid cause-and-effect relationship. One more criterion must be reached. Specifically, there can be no other viable explanation for the observed cause and effect. Researchers manipulate an independent variable and look for predicted change in a dependent variable.

But even when researchers observe an expected change in perception, attitude, or behavior following the introduction or removal of a particular environmental factor, they do not presume a cause-and-effect relationship. Only when all other possible explanations can be eliminated is a cause-and-effect statement legitimate.

Researchers eliminate alternative explanations for a cause-and-effect relationship through experimental design. They might use a control group, for example, or observe the behaviors of the same individuals before and after introducing or removing an independent variable. A research design that eliminates other possible explanations for a cause-and-effect observation is considered "internally valid."

Discussing various research designs and their associated internal validity is not our objective here. What's important to understand is this: when you conduct a root-cause analysis, significant hurdles must be jumped before you can lay claim to a legitimate cause-and-effect relationship.[13] To help you appreciate the challenge, take a look at the figure below.

Does this illustration depict a cause-and-effect relationship? In fact, the humor in the drawing is based on a self-evident root cause of the ringing in the cow's ear. The bell causes the ringing, right? But is there another possible explanation? Could other noises have caused the ringing problem? Is it possible the cow was born with the problem, or developed it over time from other noise, independent of the bell around its neck? How can we test whether the bell is the cause?

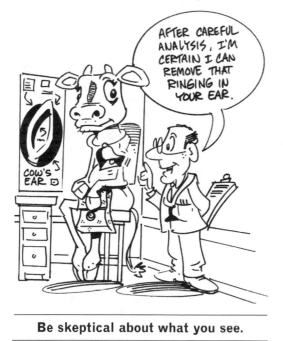

Be skeptical about what you see.

You've likely guessed one answer. Take away the bell and see if the ringing goes away. Might the ringing continue after the bell is removed? Perhaps the bell has caused permanent damage to the cow's ear, and ringing continues without the bell. Bottom line: It is not so easy to show a cause-and-effect relationship.

Skeptical researchers vs. risky safety pros

Researchers in the behavioral and social sciences are skeptical and conservative, and rarely claim they observe a cause-and-effect relationship. In contrast, it's been our experience that safety professionals in industry are quite liberal (or risky) with cause-and-effect language. They look for "root causes" of incidents, and often find what they expect to see. How? They do this through interviews, surveys, and sometimes a few behavioral observations. These are techniques insufficient at defining causal relationships.

We recall one industry safety professional claiming his organization had accomplished research that identified nine root causes of performance excellence.[14] How did they do this? While he did not detail methodology, it was evident the research was essentially based on perception surveys. The researchers obviously did not manipulate the presumed causal factors and observe change in organizational performance. Only the first of the three criteria needed to define causal factors could be achieved by the research purported to define "nine root causes."

Bottom line: We have found safety pros throughout general industry to be too cavalier with the term "root cause." They do not and cannot use the research-intensive methods needed to find a root cause. As a result, they necessarily make inaccurate or invalid assessments when looking for cause-and-effect relationships with survey, interview, and observational techniques.

If safety personnel were to assume the skeptical and conservative perspective of the researcher, they might see with more clarity the factors potentially contributing to an incident. Plus, they might broaden the spectrum of corrective action.

Inhibiting Involvement

Most importantly, a narrow-focus search for the "root cause" can lead to finding one person presumed to be responsible — the "root cause." Most staff want no part of such an "investigation" or "interrogation." Instead, the objective of an incident analysis should be to see all the various factors that could have contributed to an incident, whether it's a medication error, botched hand-off, or incorrect diagnosis.

As we have discussed, the multiple factors that contribute to an incident can be categorized as environmental, behavioral, or personal. And a comprehensive corrective action addresses each of these domains.

You need people to help you see the variety of possible factors contributing to an incident and explore the diverse array of corrective actions that could prevent another similar incident. Terminology like "possible" and "could" rather than "root cause" is not only more accurate, it enables the appropriate vision for the kind of frank and open dialogue needed for a comprehensive search of ways to reduce risks and keep patients from preventable harm.

4 The value of a systems perspective
We need a big-picture point of view

In his popular books on total quality management, *Out of the Crisis* and *The New Economics*, W. Edwards Deming tells us to focus our efforts on optimizing the system. Peter Senge stresses that "systems thinking" is the Fifth Discipline, and key to continuous improvement. And Stephen Covey's discussions of inter-dependency, win/win contingencies, and synergy in his bestseller, *The Seven Habits of Highly Effective People*, are founded on assuming a systems perspective.

How can this perspective be applied to healthcare and patient safety? Let's address this question by looking at the interplay between behaviors, attitudes, and a commitment to safety improvement.

Here's a systems perspective: You have a window seat on a flight and peer down at the maze of highways, cloverleafs, access roads, entrance and exit ramps, overpasses, bridges and tunnels that make up the transportation system circling and entwining our cities. Think of the great number of people whose driving behavior demonstrates an individualistic, win/lose attitude rather than the win/win cooperative attitude needed to optimize the system. The maze is dotted with drivers who dart back and forth between lanes, often without signaling, to shave a few seconds off their trip time. They're thinking only of themselves. It doesn't occur to them their inconsiderate, at-risk behavior could cause a crash and shut down the entire transportation system.

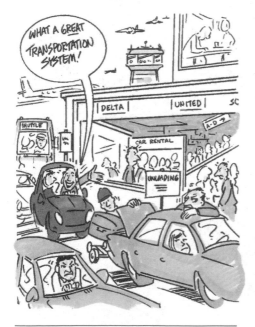

Systems thinking enables a view of the big picture.

You see slow drivers clogging up the left lane, perhaps because they'll eventually make a left-hand turn several miles ahead. They also display a win/lose perspective, perhaps unconsciously or unintentionally, which makes our transportation system less efficient.

None of these "actors" probably realize their effect on the overall system, a system that works best when everyone follows the same rules, norms, and courtesies of the road. Nor do they see the interdependency, the connection, between driving behavior and the attitudes and emotions of themselves and other drivers. Discourteous and risky driving easily triggers negative emotions in other drivers, prompting them to reciprocate with dangerous actions. It's a disruptive chain reaction.

When we see this broad interdependency between people's driving behaviors, attitudes, emotions and potential outcomes we have adopted a systems perspective. Like the view from a window seat on a plane, we need a big-picture perspective of our work situation to see the many win/win interdependencies that go into a Patient-Safety Culture. Here are seven principles that make such a perspective possible to maintain:

There is no single root cause

Don't try to find one root cause of an error or event. At-risk behavior contributes to 95 percent or more of most incidents involving harm, whether the behavior was intentional or unintentional. But this does not mean an individual's at-risk behavior is the root cause of the injury. A number of other factors are involved.

Search for environmental, behavioral, and personal factors

These factors are interactive, dynamic, and reciprocal. For example, changes in an environmental factor affect behaviors and attitudes. And behavior change usually results in some change in the environment. When people choose to change their behavior, they adjust their attitudes and beliefs (personal factors) to be consistent with their actions. This change in attitude can influence more behavior change and then more attitude change — a spiraling, reciprocal interdependency between our outward actions and inward feelings. And an initial change in behavior or attitude can be sparked by an environmental factor.

An organization's management system is one environmental factor that has dramatic impact on the human factors. A top-down authoritarian approach might dictate certain behavior, but it also creates a negative attitude that might bring about contrary behaviors.

Assess systems factors

Environmental and behavioral factors can be systematically observed with periodic audits of workplace conditions and work practices. And perception and attitude surveys can be useful barometers of person-based factors. Traditional reactive measures of safety, such as incident recordkeeping, have absolutely no diagnostic value to help understand or change system variables that cause outcomes. Keep in mind that outcome measures can be influenced by numerous factors, such as punishment and reward programs that can lead to under-reporting of incidents or close calls.

Look for facts, not faults

Because it's critical to analyze minor events and near hits, a systems perspective calls for removing any aspect of the environment that could inhibit reporting of safety-related incidents involving patients. Look for ways to facilitate the reporting and analysis of close calls and minor cases — incidents that are not typically recorded but could help prevent more serious cases.

If factors in the system promote a fault-finding perspective toward incident "investigation" (a term that implies fault-finding), then information critical to preventing harm to patients could be stifled. It's been our experience that the fault-finding perspective or "blame game" usually begins with undue focus on outcomes rather than processes.

Don't look for the quick fix

Rarely if ever does safe behavior have a built-in feedback system to support and direct it. When we take the extra time and inconvenience to protect patients from a potential risk or harm, we usually do not receive a natural consequence to motivate us to continue. (Recall the earlier discussion of Acceptable Consequences.) With a systems perspective, though, we see the bigger picture and realize that someday (if not immediately) some patient in the system will directly benefit from our effort.

Don't search for quick fixes. Cause and effect is not necessarily immediate nor linear. Taking the time to be safe today, to verify an order or double check the 5 Ps for transport — Patient, Problem, Purpose, Procedure, and Precautions — can help develop a personal habit that could pay patient-safety dividends in the future. Or it could teach others by example and protect patients now or later from errors.

Take a holistic view of your systems and you'll recognized the special need for extra feedback to motivate and activate safe behavior. The natural feedback from convenience, comfort, or a faster outcome usually competes with the completely safe way of doing something. Look for ways to support safe behavior and correct at-risk behavior. Use feedback as a consequence to motivate an individual to continue or stop a particular behavior, and as an activator to direct improvement in particular work practices.

Build consistency into your system

When we choose to do something, we experience internal pressure to maintain a personal belief system or attitude consistent with that behavior. And when we have a certain belief system or attitude toward something, such as the value of patient-safety intervention, we tend to behave in ways consistent with such beliefs or attitudes.

Researchers have found three ways to make an initial commitment to do something lead to total involvement:[15]

• First, people live up to what they write down. Ask people to commit to paper their ideas or observations regarding patient safety. Keep a log, which can be used for safety team or safety meeting discussions.

• Second, the more public the commitment, the greater the relevant attitude and behavior change, presumably because social pressures are added to the personal pressure to be consistent in word and deed. Post your patient-safety log in a place where everyone in a unit or on a floor can see who has contributed.

• Third, and perhaps most important for a public and written commitment to initiate that spiraling effect of behavior supporting attitude and vice versa, the commitment must be viewed as a personal choice. When people believe their commitment to patient safety was their idea, the consistency principle is activated. But when people believe their commitment was unduly pressured by outside forces, they don't feel a need to live up to what they were coerced to write down. This is why a number of patient-safety leaders prefer not to couch their instructions or interventions in terms of "JCAHO says…"

Build reciprocity into your system

Simply put, the reciprocity principle is reflected in the slogan, "Do for me and I'll do for you." In other words, if you're nice to someone, they'll feel obligated to return the favor. And consistent with a systems perspective, the favor might be returned to someone other than the original source.

The power of this principle can be seen at work in the interactions of effective patient-safety teams. Actively caring behavior among team members, like attentive listening, will provoke reciprocity. A person pleased to find someone actually listening to what he or she has to say will return the favor by listening attentively to someone else on the team.

People who hold true to a systems perspective see that how they react to teammates after doing them a favor can either stifle or mobilize a spiral of reci-

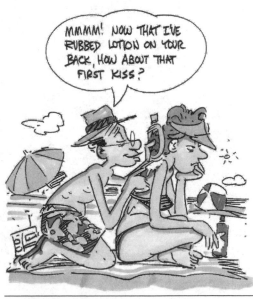

Relationships are based on reciprocity.

procity. When a person thanks someone for listening to their story, do not demean the act by saying things like, "No problem," or "It was really nothing." Anything that makes actively caring seem insignificant or trivial will reduce the impetus for reciprocity. To maintain a comfortable verbal exchange that is not belittling nor stifling, react to a "Thank you for listening" with something like, "Thank you for appreciating my effort; I know you'd do the same for me." This shows genuine admiration for the thank-you, and increases the likelihood more thanks will be given.

As you can see from these principles, the systems perspective is integral to achieving a Patient-Safety Culture. It forces us to move away from narrow views like trying to find one root cause of a near hit or injury, or focusing on outcome-based measures of performance.

The systems perspective changes our outlook from linear to circular or spiraling. Just look at the connection between activators, behaviors, and consequences. (The principle of human dynamics that serves as an underpinning of People-Based Patient Safety™.) We can see how small changes in behavior can result in attitude change, followed by more behavior change and more desired attitude change, leading eventually to personal commitment and total involvement in the process.

Ultimately, this leads to interdependent patient-safety teams and committees, and task forces regularly watching out for each other — Sentara Healthcare calls their process, "Never Leave Your Wingman" — with a win/win attitude and a proactive vision. And it all started with a systems perspective on safety.

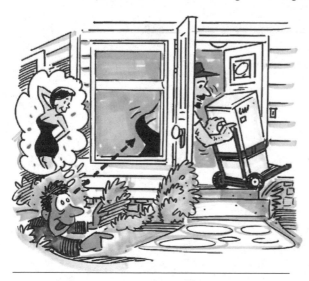

A limited view can be deceiving.

Clearly, patient-safety leaders see the big picture. "Patient-safety enthusiasts see a pathway out of the conditions in which they now work," says Julianne Morath of Children's Clinics and Hospitals of Minnesota. She says they "see" resources and solutions others in healthcare often don't know even exist — such as the performance improvement strategies and successes from other high-reliability industries, such as nuclear power and aviation.

Perception paradigms

These changes in perception are essential for developing the ultimate people-based patient system:

1) From other-directed accountability to self-directed responsibility.

2) From fault-finding to fact-finding.

3) From blaming others to asking "How can I help?"

4) From reactive score-keeping to proactive process achievement.

5) From failure-avoiding to success-seeking.

6) From being overwhelmed to feeling empowered.

7) From considering people as objects to treating people as individuals.

8) From common sense to empathic listening.

9) From the "Golden Rule" (treat others as you want to be treated) to the "Platinum Rule" (treat others as they want to be treated).

10) From win/lose independence to win/win interdependence.

5 Your patient's perspective: A valuable point of view

View the patient's experience from entry to discharge

"Why is there a need for patient-centered care? Obviously you haven't been in a hospital lately," one nurse told us. "As the patient, you are not at the center, you are not in control. You don't have an advocate. You are not communicated to decently."

Want to see where your system breaks down and puts patients at risk? "Start with the patient and work back," says Charles Inlander, president of the People's Medical Society. "Look at the patient's experience from entry to discharge from his or her point of view."

Some hospitals take a stab at this with patient surveys or "customer satisfaction" surveys. But these "exit interviews" are really another outcome measure. And as we've discussed, outcomes (or personal opinions) taken alone do not explain the ongoing activities, good or bad, that contributed to that outcome. Or in this case, what contributed to a patient's satisfied or dissatisfied opinion of his or her care.

No, you need a wide-angle perspective to understand how patients can get pushed to the side, how they are communicated to, how they lose a sense of personal control, and how they come to believe they're alone in a system they don't understand and cannot navigate. This calls for reviewing the entire process of how patients move through your healthcare system. Satisfaction surveys, on the other hand, are like those snapshots taken when customers come whooshing down the end of an amusement ride.

Shadow patients throughout their entire "ride." Time their waits for tests, and assess how long it takes for test results to reach them. Observe how tests and results are explained to patients. How much time is given for questions? Observe patient exchanges, and the exchange of verbal and written information surrounding them. How are patients' identities determined and verified as they move through your system? Is their sense of self lost through abrupt, demeaning, hurried or mechanical interactions and conversations? Or is it respected through attentive listening and open-ended questioning?

Yes, you can give every patient an exit interview. No, you can't track the experiences of every patient in this kind of detail. But you can pilot a shadowing exercise for select patients. It could be an eye-opener. Chart wait times, observe hand-offs, listen in on Q&As. Then report back to your safety team or committee. You'll share a new perspective on how your system processes patients.

A variation of this exercise in emotional intelligence — seeing experiences from another person's point of view — is when a caregiver becomes a patient. One patient-safety consultant told us: "When the doc becomes the patient, he sees the other side of all the patient-safety concerns. He becomes more appreciative of what we're trying to do."

We've also had caregivers tell us they try to provoke closer scrutiny of patient-safety practices by urging this shift in perspective: "Imagine it's your mother or your child in that bed, perhaps ready to receive the wrong dose or type of medicine. How could you not say something? How could you not 'stop the line,' regardless of negative interpersonal consequences?"

6 Don't let outcomes blind you to process activities

Patient safety is a journey, not a destination

Related to what we're saying above, there are many examples of how we can be blind to process and narrowly focused on outcome. Dr. Ellen Langer reminds us that starting in kindergarten the focus of schooling is on the final result.[16]Dr. Geller notes students in his university classes seem obsessed with their grades and seemingly lose sight of the important purpose of learning critical thinking and problem-solving skills. Likewise, travel is often seen as only a means to an end. The journey can be viewed as unimportant, just as long as the destination is reached.

Safety professionals in all industries readily see the fallacy in this logic. The way you complete a journey can determine whether you reach the destination in one piece. Orient your people to your processes — the steps needed to ensure patient safety everyday. Emphasize their involvement in deriving corrective action plans from ongoing reports of environmental/behavioral audits, near hits, case reporting.

When employees see how these successive steps or "small wins" lead to an outcome such as a reduced infection or medication error rate, their perception of mindful personal control is enhanced.

Keep tracking outcomes, of course, but make sure your staff sees the importance of discussing ongoing processes needed to prevent patient harm.

7 Stories are powerful eye openers
How to elevate a collective sense of perceived risk

If you want to elevate the collective sense of perceived risk among your staff, individual case examples are more effective than group statistics. Many people will feel a natural sympathy for vulnerable patients who suffer because of a slip or mistake. They might even vividly visualize being in the patient's place. By personalizing patients' experiences, you increase awareness and perceived risk. This suggests a shift in presentation style or content of many patient-safety meetings and training sessions. Focus on individual experiences rather than numbers.

Again we return to the critical importance of incident reporting. Your culture must encourage reporting of close calls and harmful experiences, and then discuss and otherwise disseminate those reports. When people hear the personal perceptions and regrets of harmed patients, or caregivers who made (or almost made) errors, they imagine themselves in a similar unfortunate circumstance. Their perception of risk is enhanced, and safe behavior increases.

Unfortunately, it's a simple mechanical exercise to post scores or percentages. Most organizational cultures do it, some with great fanfare. But getting people to open up and share stories that could potentially embarrass or threaten them takes more time and skill. It also requires a culture committed to eliminating selective perceptions. Effective leaders emphasize fact-finding, not fault-finding, a systems view of event investigation, and use of recognition and rewards to influence safe acting, coaching, thinking and seeing (ACTS).

8   How to peer into your culture
Dos and don'ts for conducting safety perception surveys

Want to get a reading on how your systems affect patient safety? Conduct a perception survey.

Perception surveys are useful to assess how employees see patient safety at their facilities before and after the implementation of a process to improve patient-safety-related ACTS. Pre-intervention surveys inform the design of intervention strategies, and comparisons of pre- and post-intervention surveys estimate the diverse impact of an intervention on people's perceptions, attitudes, and values.

Dr. Geller's partners in his consulting firm have been applying the same comprehensive perception survey for more than a decade, and have a database of more than 8.5 million safety-related perceptions across a broad range of industries worldwide. These culture surveys are invaluable for benchmarking, and for customizing intervention strategies for various types of operations within a particular culture.

An internet search can lead you to several downloadable surveys specific to patient safety. For example, the Agency for Healthcare Research and Quality's (AHRQ) Hospital Survey on Patient-Safety Culture is estimated to take about 10 to 15 minutes to complete and covers:
- Overall perceptions of safety
- Frequency of events reported
- Supervisor/manager expectations and actions promoting patient safety
- Organizational learning and continuous improvement
- Teamwork within units
- Communication transparency
- Feedback about errors
- Nonpunitive response to error
- Staffing

A word of caution: "Conducting a perception survey on patient safety 'is no slam dunk' in many organizations," says Cynthia Barnard, director of quality strategies for Northwestern Memorial Hospital in Chicago.

For one thing, data-driven managers don't trust barometers of feelings. "Paul O'Neill (former Alcoa chairman, U.S. Treasury secretary and now an active patient-safety proponent) was here and he wanted to talk about the number of events," says one hospital administrator. "His view was, 'Show me results, not culture surveys.'"

That perception is widely held in industry, we can tell you from experience — and from surveys. Asked to rank the significance of eight safety and health tools, safety professionals responding to a 2003 survey[17] scored perception surveys dead last. Only 13 percent considered them important tools.

What's the problem?

People have a tendency to ignore or dither over results, for one thing. Survey tabs are often never analyzed or used for interventions. Dr. Geller recalls visiting a client who had "gobs and gobs of paper, reams of paper from a perception survey. He threw up his hands and cried, 'Now what?'"

A bigger barrier is fear. Recalls a safety manager in the chemical industry: "I was in charge of developing a case for safety perception surveys at my corporation when we launched our response to a major disaster in the early '90s. After I brought in a leading consultant to perform the studies, and the implications of what was going to happen were fully realized by management, the project was cancelled. It was clear that getting unbiased input from the rank and file to determine how safe they felt, and whether they felt they had the tools to perform at a 'world-class safety level' was going to create and unleash extremely powerful forces that management would not be able to fully control. Management's realization of that loss of control led to the immediate demise of the project."[18]

Delivering on the promise

OK, so how do you realize the promise of perception surveys? How do you develop surveys that can lead to goals, plans and culture-enrichment?

Here are steps you can take:

• Form a multi-disciplinary perception survey design team consisting of management, caregivers and non-medical employee reps. Be up-front about those fears mentioned earlier, point out the hazards of sticking your head in the sand. Search the internet using a "patient-safety perception survey" to find case studies of how other healthcare systems have used surveys, and what surveys are available. It's your call whether to bring in consulting expertise or network and do it yourself.

• Agree on the survey design, content, and delivery method. Keep it simple. You don't need to ask 99 questions. Design your questions to be remedial. Each question should tackle a patient-safety issue that can be fixed by managers and frontline staff working together.

• Announce and promote your survey. Sell the troops hard. Reassure them it's OK to criticize. It's OK to talk about things that haven't been brought up before.

• Tell your folks this is not about whining or hurling grenades at mahogany row. Focus your questions on what affects communications, teamwork, reporting, risk abatement and other patient-safety issues on a day-to-day level.

• Don't pressure those who don't want to participate.

• Survey a sufficient number of people to ensure representativeness. Make sure survey responses reflect a cross-section of all levels of your organization.

• Make sure employee participation is anonymous. Use credible, respected coworkers — your "social influencers" and patient-safety leaders — to help market the survey and give it positive word-of-mouth.

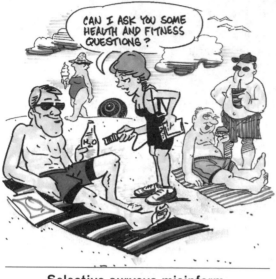

Selective surveys misinform.

• When you review results, accept that some suggestions will be off the wall. Keep feedback from veering into petty, impractical areas. And be sure to explain why some suggestions are irrelevant or not feasible.

• Look at bottom line total responses for the questions you've posed. Also, compare answers from managers, supervisors, and workers. Look for obvious gaps in perceptions, such as disconnects between the floor and the front office.

Industrial safety expert Dan Petersen once analyzed perception survey data from 56 companies employing a total of 1.6 million people. He concluded a score below 70 percent positive for a category (say the effectiveness of safety training) at the staff level suggested a need to examine activities in that area. A score below 60 percent positive was a red flag that an organizational function was faltering.[19]

In Petersen's comprehensive analysis, the most common problems in general industry safety programs turned up in the areas of recognition for performance — "Is good safety performance recognized at all levels of the organization?" — (56.9 percent positive) and discipline — "Is the company perceived as taking a fair approach to handling rules and infractions?" — (58.4 percent positive).[20]

• Publicize your survey results. Feed results back especially to those employees who took the survey.

• Assemble task groups for problem-solving. These can be focus groups of employees, supers and managers who crunch numbers and interpret scores. Develop an action plan with timelines. Plans must be reviewed by senior managers, and implemented with their clear support. Managers should hold assigned individuals accountable for implementing the plan and meeting deadlines.

• Monitor what happens next. By all means follow up. Chart changes using activity measures (number of training sessions conducted, risks identified and mitigated, etc.) and repeat the perception survey every year or two.

Changes to watch for over time are:
- Increased participation at patient-safety meetings.
- Frontline staff demonstrating more active respect for patient safety, perhaps through greater use of gloves and respirators when called for, more handwashing, greater use of tools such as the START checklist and SBAR during hand-offs.
- Staff are more willing to give and take feedback on patient-safety matters.
- Increased reporting of observed adverse events, close calls and risks.
- Managers and supervisors visibly demonstrating the importance of patient safety, and holding subordinates accountable for their patient-safety performance.

Expert Q&A *Safety culture surveys*

Cynthia Barnard, MBA, MSJS, CPHQ, is director of quality strategies at Northwestern Memorial Hospital in Chicago, Illinois, where she is responsible for patient safety, accreditation and licensure, patient satisfaction measurement, and medical ethics. She can be reached at cbarnard@nmh.org.

Q *What has been your experience with patient-safety culture surveys as improvement tools?*

A *Most hospitals aren't using anything at this point, or they are relying on employee satisfaction surveys and engagement surveys. (We use Gallup's Q12 survey for our evaluation of employee engagement.) Some culture assessment is done implicitly through observation rounds and analyzing complaints or certain outcomes. But the vast majority of hospitals are doing nothing yet.*

Why? Different factors are at work. Getting acceptance of culture surveys is no slam dunk. Culture surveys are still too new a topic. Although it seems intuitively clear culture will affect patient safety on every level, there is not much solid evidence or published research yet. In addition, clinicians can be extremely skeptical of a survey's "soft" data. Some will dismiss anything which seems so subjective. Since there's no clear mandate for culture surveying, it doesn't rise to the top of the list of things to do. Many hospitals will work on improving incident reporting or other clearly useful tactical improvements instead.

At this organization, we created our own patient-safety culture survey in 2002. We wanted to assess general areas of potential opportunity. The survey yielded a very limited response rate and appeared to reflect a mildly positive culture, but was not very actionable. When AHRQ (the Agency for Healthcare Research and Quality) released its patient-safety culture survey in 2004, we immediately implemented it to develop valid baseline data in preparation for targeted interventions. We wanted pre- and post-intervention data to see what effects we could identify. Senior management here believes in the importance of culture, and felt we needed a good barometer of our status and future progress.

We pilot-tested a survey with a focus group of physicians, pharmacists, and nurses. One thing we learned was docs were a bit confused by the term "supervisor" in the standard AHRQ survey questions. We had been concerned about the AHRQ survey length, but our pilot demonstrated it took only about 10 to 12 minutes to answer the questions.

We implemented the AHRQ tool as an online email survey to 8,000 employees, everyone in the institution. The non-clinical people generally did not respond, which was fine, since the survey really is focused on clinicians' experiences. (If we had a better way to distribute the survey only to clinical staff, we would have done so, but we did not have that capability.) We allowed about one month for responses to come in, and we sent out two email reminders. We received 1,654 valid responses from an estimated 5,000 persons eligible. We felt that was a decent response rate, though of course there are no benchmarks for this yet.

What did we learn? The AHRQ survey poses safety questions in different domains, so you can learn what your people think about communications, reporting, management support, exchanges and hand-offs, work climate and teamwork, for example. You can assess results by clinical area, by staff position, and by years of experience. (We elected not to ask respondents to identify a specific nursing unit, to preserve anonymity this first time. We do not have data to analyze results by unit, but we can analyze perceptions by area such as medicine, surgery, operating rooms, emergency department, etc.)

We had about twice as many nurses respond as physicians. We found that nurses and physicians generally agreed the least positive domain in terms of patient safety was hand-offs and transitions of care. This was completely consistent with our expectations and analytic work, based on observation rounds.

Nurses were very positive regarding teamwork within units, but less positive regarding teamwork across departments. Again, this had a lot of face validity based on all our patient-safety analysis and improvement work, and provided more evidence this survey was identifying valid and meaningful themes for our hospital.

An important outcome of the survey was to increase our focus on communicating what we are doing in patient safety hospital-wide. Physician ratings indicated their concerns about not getting enough feedback and communication about errors. We give a great deal of feedback to nurses; it's easier because nurses are employees, they come to staff meetings, and they get regular feedback from their managers. It's more difficult to provide this feedback to 1,200 physicians and more than 800 residents and fellows, and the survey results were helpful in identifying this as an area requiring improvement.

Since mid-2004, we've held monthly interdisciplinary patient-safety morbidity and mortality conferences for all interested staff (physicians, nurses, pharmacists, all clinical and support staff) in which we go through actual cases and perform a mini-root-cause analysis. Since the AHRQ survey, we've worked harder to communicate the availability of these rounds and attendance has improved. In addition, we've encouraged individual medical staff departments to use cases we can provide to them in their own departmental M&M conferences. We develop summaries based on actual events or near-miss events at our own hospital, or from significant cases in the literature.

We also worked to improve feedback for nurses; for example, a written patient-safety M&M case is written up every month for nurse managers and their staff to review and provide their recommendations. With about 1,600 nurses, it's helpful to have different communication methods.

In general we've become much more candid talking about patient safety and what we are doing, and need to do, to improve the safety of our systems. We are always looking for ways to listen to the clinicians' concerns and ideas. It certainly is a challenge to build these communications with physicians, nurses and other important clinicians.

The AHRQ survey has been quite successful for us. It yielded a wonderful response rate, and the results both validated our general impressions about appropriate areas for focus, and emphasized the importance to work on those and others. It established a baseline from which we plan to measure approximately every 18 months. The survey has the advantage of clarity, comprehensiveness, and technical validation, and we are looking forward to the AHRQ's eventual plan to offer some benchmarking.

9 You must see past denial
"We really didn't know how big a problem we had..."

From global and local perspectives, healthcare has had the blinders on when it comes to patient safety. One nurse calls it "125 years of denial and complacency."

To be sure, all systems are susceptible to myopia. In the case of healthcare, "the CEO says patient safety is not a problem in my facility. The doctor says patient safety is not a problem in my practice," says Ilene Corina, founder of PULSE, a patient-safety advocacy group. Her words reflect a culture of compartmentalization, where adverse events usually are isolated and individually experienced. For any one physician working in his/her sphere, medical errors indeed may seem infrequent, says one physician.

"People have always been worried about patient safety, but we really did not know how big a problem we had until we researched it," says Lori Paine, patient safety coordinator for The Johns Hopkins Hospital.

Getting people to be reflective about safety is fundamental to developing a Patient-Safety Culture, says Dr. Jeff Cooper, director of biomedical engineering for Partners Healthcare System.

Administering perception surveys is like holding a mirror to a culture. If you looked yourself in the mirror, how would you grade out on the ACTS continuum of patient- safety-related actions, coaching, thinking and seeing? You might also want to look at how your personality affects your perceptions of risk and patient safety. Dr. Geller relates how "my Type-A personality and need-to-achieve attitude facilitate a future-oriented perspective that gives too much attention to the future and too little on the present."

"But I'm working hard at perceiving and seizing the moment," he promises. That means being mindful and attentive to ongoing behavior in every respect. Using all relevant senses to recognize what you are doing and where you are doing it. It's a perceptual orientation that surely makes a mishap unlikely.

It's surely preferable to the perspective described in *Internal Bleeding*: "Doctors and nurses get caught in their own procedural and cognitive quicksand, put on blinders, and see nothing but those things that reinforce their previous judgments and beliefs."[21]

10 Beware of technology blind spots
System improvements might lower perceptions of risk

When you feel protected, do you take more risks? Many people do. Such increased risk-taking is due to perception. People presumably accept a certain

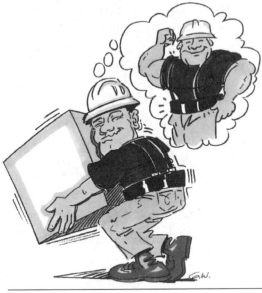

level of risk, which varies widely across individuals. This perception is influenced by a number of factors, from personality characteristics to prior training and experience. When their perception of risk changes, people change their behavior accordingly. Psychologists call it risk compensation or risk homeostasis.[22]

One particular implication of this phenomenon is worth noting: improving patient safety with system enhancements (computerized physician order entry and medication bar coding, to name two) might actually lower staff risk perception — and unintentionally lead to an increase in risky behavior.

It's important to note this change in perception and behavior as a function of protection is intu-

Perception is not reality.

itive (we all let our guard down when we feel more secure) and is supported with sound research, but it has not been specifically validated in healthcare settings regarding technology. Still, we think it is prudent for patient-safety coaches, leaders and teams to be aware of what might happen to risk perceptions when new technology or controls are introduced. Consider this 2005 press report:[23]

Computerized Physician-Order Entry Systems Often Facilitate Medication Errors

Philadelphia, PA – Healthcare policymakers and administrators have championed specialty-designed software systems — including the highly-touted Computerized Physician Order Entry (CPOE) systems — as the cornerstone of improved patient safety. CPOE systems are claimed to significantly reduce medication-prescribing errors. "Our data indicate that that is often a false hope," said sociologist Ross Koppel, Ph.D., of the Center for Clinical Epidemiology and Biostatistics at the University of Pennsylvania School of Medicine.

"Good computerized physician order entry systems are, indeed, very helpful and hold great promise; but, as currently configured, there are at least two dozen ways in which CPOE systems significantly, frequently, and commonly facilitate errors — and some of those errors can be deadly," said Koppel.

Koppel and colleagues studied the day-to-day medication-ordering patterns and interactions of house staff working in a tertiary-care teaching hospital, which at that time, ran a popular CPOE system. In addition to a comprehensive survey of almost 90 percent of the house staff who use CPOE, the researchers also shadowed the doctors and pharmacists, as well as performed interviews with the hospital's attending physicians, nurses, IT and pharmacy leaders, and administrators. As a result, they identified 22 discreet ways in which medication-errors were facilitated by the CPOE system they studied. Findings were published in the *Journal of the American Medical Association.*

Koppel and his research team grouped error types into two main categories: information errors and human-machine interface flaws. Information errors, explained Koppel, result from fragmentation of data and information, or when there is a failure to fully integrate a hospital's multiple computer and information systems.

Examples: A physician orders the wrong dose of a drug because the CPOE system displays pharmacy warehouse information that is misinterpreted by the physician as clinical-dosage guidelines. Or warnings about antibiotics are placed in the paper chart and not seen by physicians who are using only the computerized system.

Human-machine interface flaws reflect machine rules that do not correspond to organizational routines or usual work behaviors. For example, within the CPOE system studied, Koppel's research team found that up to 20 screens might be needed to view the totality of just one patient's medications — thereby increasing the risk of selecting a wrong medication.

Bar coding caveats

Similar words of caution emerged from a 2001 study of side effects from a natural experiment, the implementation of bar code medication administration (BCMA), a technology designed to reduce adverse drug events (ADEs).[24]

Researchers identified five negative side effects after BCMA implementation: (1) nurses confused by automated removal of medications by BCMA; (2) degraded coordination between nurses and physicians; (3) nurses dropping activities to reduce workload during busy periods; (4) increased prioritization of monitored activities during goal conflicts; and (5) decreased ability to deviate from routine sequences.[25]

Breakdowns between nurses and physicians caught our eye. The study noted: "During the observations, numerous coordination breakdowns occurred between nurses and physicians, some of which might not have occurred with the previous paper-based system. Prior to BCMA, physicians were observed to have quick access at the bedside to current medication administration information and nurses had immediate access to information about pending and discontinued orders on their paper medication administration record (MAR).[26]

"…In a focus group conducted October 26, 2001, seven of seven residents stated they did not systematically look at a patient's medication orders in BCMA unless a question was asked because it is a time-intensive process. In comparison, they estimated that with a paper-based system at another hospital, they reviewed the medication orders for each patient an average of 3 times/week."[27]

Cautioned the researchers: "These side effects might create new paths to ADEs. We recommend design revisions, modification of organizational policies, and 'best practices' training that could potentially minimize or eliminate these side effects before they contribute to adverse outcomes."[28]

11 Universal perceptions of change
Quickly respond to "What's in it for me?"

Everyone tunes into radio station WIIFM — What's In It For Me? So let's talk about six universal perceptions of employees when a new process or procedure is introduced — such as a patient-safety roll-out. If you anticipate and deal quickly with the critical views your frontline staff has about change, it's possible to launch a new patient-safety initiative with more participants and fewer resisters.

Why is the change needed?
This is perhaps the most obvious issue to address, but it's often overlooked. Why is the new approach better than the old way? This is a matter of education — explaining the rationale, theory, or principles behind the change.

And if the new approach is dictated by a JCAHO patient-safety requirement, please offer benefits beyond compliance. Numerous patient-safety leaders tell us they refrain from framing patient-safety initiatives in terms of "JCAHO says…" Recall the perceptual bias that framing produces. When it comes to lecturing on externally derived rules, the bias morphs into what one nurse described as the "robot glaze."

Remember, there's a difference between "education" and "training." Training programs that only teach step-by-step safety procedures or cling to accreditation requirements can be perceived as a top-down "flavor of the month." Educating people about the principles or rationale behind a new safety policy, program or process enables understanding and critical thinking. It also allows you to customize procedures for particular work situations.

What's in it for me?
Don't let your people speculate on how a particular change will affect them. Be honest about the extra effort or adjustment involved in making the change work, and emphasize the positive consequences that can be expected. If you can't define positive gains and/or negative consequences avoided due to the new process, you'll have a difficult time motivating participation. So it's important to clarify the costs and benefits of any new program or process.

What will I have to do?

People want to know what they will need to do differently. Do they have the knowledge, skills, and resources to accomplish their role in your change effort? It's important to convince potential participants the new responsibilities are within their capabilities. If they don't currently have the ability to perform these tasks competently, assure them they will be taught relevant procedures.

Who else will be involved?

This question targets issues of collaboration and teamwork, and personal versus interpersonal control. Does the success of the new process depend on input from others inside and outside the microsystem of a unit culture? From people we don't know, or people we have little influence over?

Spell out the degree of coordination and cooperation needed for success. If interdependent support is needed, suggest ways to make it happen. Remember, if success hinges on cooperation from people in different units, individual participants will perceive they have little personal control over the outcome, and will be more uncertain of success.

How will my participation be evaluated?

People are naturally concerned about accountability. Everyone wants to know how their performance will be judged. Employees want to participate competently in worthwhile endeavors, but their feelings of competence are influenced by the methods used to observe and rank performance.

Be prepared to answer these questions: "Will the external measure of competence be objective?" "How much of my effectiveness score will be determined by factors outside my personal control?" "If we feel an evaluation is unfair, can we suggest another approach?"

Can we suggest improvements?

If you convince your audience specific patient-safety improvements are called for and their individual participation is needed, you should anticipate suggestions for customizing and refining the new process.

In fact, you might skip giving specific step-by-step procedural instructions completely, unless spelled out in a requirement. Instead, give your vision for breakthrough improvement (or the stated objective of a patient-safety requirement, if that's the impetus for change) and a general structure or set of guidelines for accomplishing the desired change. Leave plenty of room for individuals and work teams to derive specific procedures.

Keep in mind many accreditation-related patient-safety objectives use language such as, "create and use a process…" "implement a process for…" or "implement a standardized approach to…" JCAHO allows for demonstrations of the effectiveness of alternative approaches. (The form and instructions for submitting alternative approaches are available on the Joint Commission website.) Tailoring a process to one's own work area spurs creativity and owner-ship — and also provides the most suitable procedures for a particular situation.

It's important to encourage continuous refinement of a new safety process. When people perceive competence at performing a task they believe is worth-while, they will develop new and better ways to succeed. Make it clear from the start this is expected.

12 How to ease sensory overload
Free up abilities to recognize risks

Eliminate signs, slogans, exhortations, and objectives from the workplace, W. Edwards Deming told us.[29] Did he mean we ought to stop giving people direc-tions to follow, goals to shoot for? If he did, he was denying the basic activator-behavior-consequence framework for behavior-based patient safety we discussed in Chapters 2 and 3. Substantial research has verified that behavior is influenced markedly by activators (like signs preceding behavior) and by consequences (pleasant or unpleasant events following behavior).[30]

We don't think Dr. Deming was telling us to stop looking at signs and slogans. Rather, he was criticizing the standard top-down development and display of performance activators. As currently used for safety, they might only raise expectations without giving relevant and meaningful direction. If that's the case, we might was well gaze right past them.

Consider these six guidelines for increasing the impact of visual activa-tors.

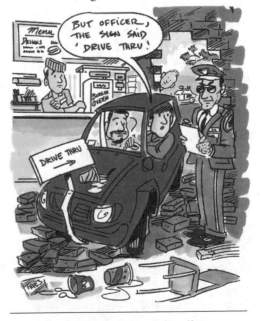

Some signs are misleading.

Get specific
Signs that refer to a specific behavior can be beneficial. Don't expect signs or slogans that urge employees to "Think Safe," "Eliminate Accidents," or "Achieve Zero Infections" to do much good. More effective are messages that alert employees — "Hand-washing required," "Designated Non-Smoking Area," and "Radiation Exposure" — or instruct, such as "Lift

With Legs," "Remove metal objects," and "Buckle Up for Safety." Note, too, these signs are not overly complex.

Avoid complacency

It is perfectly natural for sign messages to lose their impact over time. It's human nature to habituate, or no longer see, everyday activators in our environment that are not supported by some consequence. This is the case with many safety activators. A sign requesting compliance with CDC hand-hygiene guidelines might eventually be ignored, for example, if consequences (positive feedback or penalties) are not in place to support the message.

Vary the message

Over the years we've noticed a variety of techniques for changing the message on safety signs, such as removable slats to place different messages and computer-generated signs with an infinite variety of safety messages. In industry, some plants hang video monitors in break areas, lunch rooms, visitor lounges, and hallways that display many kinds of safety messages. The same people expected to follow these specific messages should have as much input as possible in defining their content.

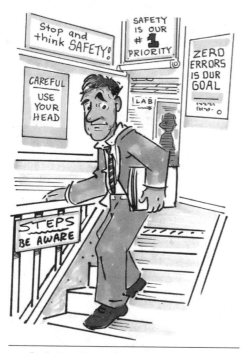

Safety signs without behavioral directions are overload.

Involve the workforce

When public trash receptacles include the logos of nearby businesses, the merchants whose logos are displayed typically take care of the receptacle, and keep the surrounding area clean. Consider the success of "Adopt-a-Highway" programs that have groups keep a certain roadway clear of litter and perhaps beautified with plants, shrubs, or flowers. The same sense of commitment is possible in a workplace.

Carefully consider placement

A safety message placed in the work area where the behavior it specifies is to occur has greater impact than putting the same message in an email, newsletter, or as a pop-up on a computer screen. It's like "point-of-purchase advertising" — placing ads at locations where the target products can be purchased.[31]

"Deliver information at the point of use, such as on soap dispensers" says Peter Perreiah, managing director of the Pittsburgh Regional Healthcare

Initiative. He recalls healthcare workers in one unit with chapped and cracked skin on their hands because different types of soap were not labeled. The physical arrangement of visual cues can't be overlooked as a factor determining whether or not directions are seen and followed, he says.

Similarly, road signs that gave drivers feedback on the percentage of vehicles exceeding posted speed limits have been found through research to be more effective at reducing speeding than public service announcements on radio and television.[32]

Specify consequences

Activators are most potent when they refer to internal (self-imposed) or external consequences — in terms of incentives and disincentives.

One last point: We really don't need more messages telling us what to do in our lives. We're already bombarded at work and at home by information. We should plan our messages so they receive the attention and ultimate action they deserve.

(13) How to recognize & assess risk
Prioritize hazards based on exposure, severity and probability

Hospitals are self-contained communities where people are born and die, live and work, sleep and eat, come and go. They have their own transport and power systems, their own sanitation and food services. And like any city, hospitals harbor an incredible array of risks. To name just a few possible environmental hazards that can threaten patient safety:

- Wet floors
- Broken alarm settings for telemetry and bedside monitoring systems
- Wheelchairs with malfunctioning brakes
- Heating pads, microwavable hot packs, and hot-water bottles that can cause burns
- Broken safety latches for needles
- Medical devices — like the gel pack in a defibrillator — used after the labeled expiration date
- Unlabeled containers
- Torn mattress or wheelchair covers that can harbor deadly microorganisms
- Contaminated equipment.

In light of the perceptual biases and filters we've described, how do you make sure staff sees and responds to the most serious risks present?

Prioritize.

First, recall from our discussion of the Safety Triad, risks may be environmental in nature (a broken wheelchair), behavioral (continued use of a broken wheelchair), or arise from what we call person states (an impulsive and rushing nurse forces a patient to walk instead of taking extra time to fetch a wheelchair).

It's most easy to audit for environmental risks. Brainstorm in a team or patient-safety meeting what those risks might be within a unit, and draw up a checklist for making environmental scanning rounds.

For behavioral risks, customize a critical behavior checklist (CBC). Recall from Chapter 2 on Acting, the CBC consists of a list of specific behaviors required to complete a task or procedure safely. Observers distinguish and give feedback on "safe" and "at-risk" actions. Definitions of "safe" versus "at-risk" are developed through structured group discussions and consensus building.

Don't take the development of a CBC lightly. When you decide what safety-related behaviors are "critical," you define aspects of a job that require the most attention and mindfulness. These are the behaviors people will hold each other accountable to perform safely.

Sources for deciding which behaviors to include on a CBC include:
• Reports from daily rounds
• Morbidity & mortality conferences
• Patient-safety perception surveys
• Interviews with patients
• Root-cause analyses
• Open-ended incident narratives
• Near-hit reports
• Patient-safety operating procedures
• Accreditation requirements
• Outcome measures relating to patient safety which can be traced back for frontline contributing factors.

Talk to your staff.

Employees already know a lot about their own safe and at-risk work practices. They know which safety rules are ignored. They know when a near-hit or close call has happened to them or to others due to at-risk behavior.

As for risks that stem from internal person states — possibly fatigue, substance abuse, perceptual biases, mental shortcuts, memory lapses, burnout, personality traits or states — we emphasize the word "possibly."

Resist the temptation to play counselor.

Not everyone is qualified, either by stature, authority, the nature of a working relationship, or interpersonal communication skills, to engage in what the book, *Complications*, describes as the "Terribly Quiet Chat."[33]Every culture tends to have its variation of the chat, where close associates privately express concerns, gently or bluntly, to an apparently wayward peer. Sometimes this approach can work.[34] But adverse reactions can easily be the outcome: denials, arguments, attempts to find defenders.

Don't try to peer inside someone's head. Follow protocols for dealing with disruptive, erratic or otherwise at-risk behavior if they are available, or avail yourself of employee assistance expertise.

Evaluating exposure, severity and probability

Once risks are identified, we consider three factors: exposure, severity and probability. Imagine all risks on a severity scale. At the top are the most serious, the ones with the most potential to cause patient injury or death. At the bottom are less serious risks, those you can attend to after you deal with the most serious threats to patients. This is how we come up with a step-by-step plan for what to focus on first, then next, and on and on.

Discuss each of these dimensions of risk within a group or in a meeting to facilitate developing and refining your risk recognition practices.

Exposure: Every time an at-risk behavior occurs relevant to patient safety, a patient somewhere in the system is exposed to potential harm. The threat could be immediate or delayed. The more often this behavior occurs and the more people performing it, the greater the exposure — more patients may be harmed. For example, misreading a prescription order is a serious enough risk, potentially even a fatal one, if done even once. Now multiply this risk by a physician with notoriously bad handwriting who writes out thousands of orders and you gain a different perspective.

Severity: You might ask: What's the worst that could happen here? If it's a behavioral risk, like allowing a patient to fall out of bed, there could be serious physical injuries that complicate recovery. If it's an environmental hazard like a spill on the floor, patients could slip getting out of bed even if they were not considered a fall risk.

Probability: What's the probability a risk will result in harm? This is a subjective judgment, the most difficult risk assessment to make. Consider a wheelchair with faulty brakes. By counting the daily opportunities to transport patients using this wheelchair, you can get a good estimate of exposure. It's not hard to imagine the worst possible outcome of a severe crash.

But how probable is it a wheelchair with faulty brakes (let's say they are balky and require strong hand pressure to operate safely) will cause a crash and harm of any severity? Many factors come into play — the age and physical strength of both the transporter and the patient, the duration and destination of the transport. When the transporter is aware the wheelchair has ineffective braking, he can compensate, or simply refuse to use the chair. In this case, the probability of harm to a patient decreases. But what if the transporter is rushed and forgets? This is what makes probability such an unpredictable assessment.

Using ESP

You can remember the three characteristics used to estimate relative risk — exposure, severity, and probability of occurrence — as the "ESP approach."

Exposure fluctuates according to the frequency and duration of the at-risk behavior or environmental condition faced by the patients. It is the easiest of the three risk factors to estimate.

Severity is judged by visualizing the worst possible consequence that could happen to a patient from the at-risk behavior or condition.

Probability is most difficult to estimate because so many environmental and individual factors influence the likelihood of an at-risk behavior or environmental hazard resulting in patient harm. As with severity, a conservative approach is recommended. Assume bad luck, meaning all the factors that could increase the possibility of harm are in place, from unfriendly environmental conditions to an individual whose attention periodically deviates from the task.

Using the "worst-case scenario" is one way to evaluate risks to a patient's safety:

STEP 1: Exposure/High – Medium – Low — How often is this patient exposed to that potential risk/hazard and for how long?

STEP 2: Severity/High – Medium – Low — How badly could the patient be injured as a result of exposure to this risk/hazard?

STEP 3: Probability/High – Medium – Low — How likely is it that taking the risk could cause injury — or death?

If the exposure, severity and probability all score high, you're dealing with a hazard that demands immediate attention and continuous monitoring. When the risk is lower, immediate attention is not as critical.

When we use the hazard assessment scale and techniques like scanning and focusing, we can overcome the blind spots and hazard recognition traps.

14   How to scan & focus
Overcoming daily diversions

Dr. Geller was flying to Erie, Pennsylvania to present a safety workshop. After landing, he took a cab to his hotel. Along the way he called in for messages, but was interrupted when the cabbie started asking him about the Virginia Tech football team.

Dr. Geller put down his cell phone and talked Hokies football until reaching the hotel. In his room, he reached in his backpack for his cell phone to get back to those messages. Guess what? It wasn't there. He called the cab driver, and sure enough, the phone was in the back seat.

The following night Dr. Geller returned home and got to his car at the Roanoke, Virginia airport about 11:30 p.m., only to find a dead battery. The headlight switch had been "accidentally" turned on. He eventually located a battery charger, but without a flashlight he couldn't find the positive and negative labels on the battery poles. What he thought was the black cover to the negative pole was not. Guess what? He fried his battery, and blew a main fuse. At 2:00 a.m., he was being towed 40 miles to Blacksburg, Virginia.

Daily diversions

Yes, these glitches illustrate the critical role of attention in accomplishing everyday routines — and how easily our attention can be diverted and lead to at-risk behavior and negative consequences. Plus, it's not enough simply knowing how important attention is to safely accomplishing activities.

Awareness of "inattentional blindness" — a term coined by psychologists who have studied people's inability to detect unexpected objects in their field of vision when their attention is focused elsewhere[35] — is just the start. What can we do about this potential cause of an injury?

Obviously, changing our attentional focus can remove the "blinders." But this is easier said than done. When we're busy, it's annoying to divert attention elsewhere. But this is a recommended intervention. When focusing on details, step back intermittently and take a wider view of the situation. Scan for possible risks and safety-related consequences. Competent workers know where to focus their attention and what to tune out. They also know when to take a wide-angle view of their environment. We call this "scanning."

Plan to scan

Some tasks require more scanning than focusing. Take driving, for example. Sustained focus on one aspect of driving is quite risky, say when you're punching in numbers on your cell phone. Competent drivers shift their attention: from the road and oncoming traffic to vehicles beside and behind them; and they occasionally check the speedometer. They continually scan the visual fields observed through their windshield, side windows, and rear-view mirror.

Lack of periodic scanning or excessive focusing can put patients at risk. Errors and near-errors can be caused by narrowly focused attention without sufficient environmental scanning. Here's a hypothetical example: A patient is crashing, and the physician, respiratory therapist and ER nurse rush to intubate him. But the team doesn't immediately see that his blood pressure has dropped to a dangerously low level on the monitor. The team was so fixated on the problem, they lost sight of the big picture. They didn't notice the monitor and the significant change in vital signs. If the team had alternately scanned the environment, then refocused on the intubation procedure, they would have noticed his blood pressure was unstable.

It's often critical to vary attention from scanning to focusing. Developing a critical behavior checklist should include discussing when and how often to scan versus focus visual attention while performing a particular task. A CBC is a good coaching tool to increase the kinds of ongoing attention strategies we need in the workplace.

FAQ *Perception survey tools are increasingly popular in building and identifying weaknesses in patient safety cultures. Do you have any caveats to offer regarding the use of these surveys?*

Perception surveys are critical to evaluating people's opinions and attitudes regarding healthcare. They can be given to healthcare deliverers or receivers. They should be given periodically to assess change. In other words, a perception survey measures changeable states not immutable traits. Therefore, it is necessary to assess perceptions periodically if there is interest in continuous improvement.

Reliability and validity issues are always relevant when perception surveys are used for research. Reliability means the survey is consistent and will give the same results at another time. This is analogous to stepping on a scale to measure weight on a series of days and getting the same weight. In contrast, validity is more complex and reflects a number of concepts, including consistency with theory, ability to predict future behavior, and discrimintability. In my opinion, these research concepts are beyond the scope of applying perception surveys in healthcare settings.

The challenge is to customize a series of questions related to perceptions to assess. "Yes" versus "no" choices following a series of questions is less desirable than asking for a numerical rating between "1" (for completely disagree) to "7" (for completely agree). Such a numerical score is more sensitive and thereby can reflect change more regularly. Because perception surveys measure states, scores can vary from one time to the next. And, different people will provide different perception scores. Reliability can be estimated from statistics that measure inter-item consistency within the perception scale. Also, a factor analysis can be conducted to determine the number of independent factors or perception domains assessed by a particular perception survey. This kind of analysis typically requires consultation from a program evaluator or statistician, and is really not necessary for an ongoing assessment of healthcare perceptions.

Bottom line: I recommend using perception surveys rather loosely. In other words, you need not be concerned with reliability and validity from a research perceptive. Consider the development and application of perception surveys a ongoing learning experience. You not only learn people's attitudes and opinions about specific protocol or healthcare events/issues, you also learn how to develop informative questions. In other words, you should be open to altering and adding questions on subsequent perception surveys after studying a perception survey.

One important point: perception surveys can benefit from open ended questions. Consider, for example, asking patients the following three questions: 1) What did you like best about your treatment at this facility? 2) What was the least desirable aspect of your treatment by caretakers at this facility? 3) What specifically could be improved regarding the caretaking at this facility? These three questions are just examples. I recommend customizing a few open-ended questions to fit your particular needs.

FAQ *Is there one perceptual "trap" that stands out as really needing to be addressed first and foremost?*

The most serious perceptual bias is premature cognitive commitment. Of course, this includes a broad range of biases. Anything that prejudices perception can be detrimental to patient safety. An individual's past experiences including prior education and family upbringing, influences perceptions and therefore attitudes and behavior.

Ideal health workers are flexible and open to new perspectives. They are not stuck in the past with traditional approaches to patient safety. They are open to learning new ways to improving the safety of their patients. They consider their

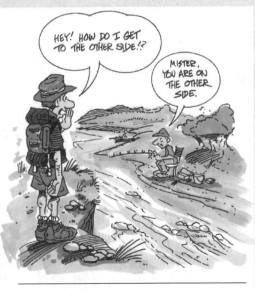

Two different people have two different perspectives.

job an opportunity to learn and improve. Indeed, their healthcare culture is a learning organization.

CHAPTER 6 *Keeping It Going*

In this chapter you'll learn 8 essentials of sustainability:

1 Leadership

You don't "manage" to build a culture

We've watched general industry try to "manage" safety, to varying degrees of success for more than 30 years. And now, as patient safety moves more to the center of healthcare management's radar screen, it's worth distinguishing safety management from safety leadership. What we've learned is this: an organization can and must "manage" safety issues day-to-day; you can "manage" compliance every day, for instance. But you don't "manage" to build a culture of safety. Leadership is required.

You see, leaders help build self-directed responsibility for safety. And a culture of safety is comprised of individuals, ultimately every employee in the organization, taking personal responsibility for safety — more specifically, patient safety as it relates here.

This is not meant to belittle management or even to suggest we need less management. We only want to stress that to build and sustain a patient-safety culture, you need to apply both management and leadership skills. Here's how those skills match up:

Focus

Managers are typically held accountable for numbers, and they use outcome numbers to motivate safety performance. But as we've discussed earlier, these scores and percentages, are reactive, reflect failure, and are not diagnostic for prevention.

Safety leaders hold people accountable for accomplishing activities that can prevent patient harm. When people see improvement in the process numbers — incident reports filed and analyzed; patient-safety risks identified and "fixed" — they are reinforced for their efforts and develop a sense of personal responsibility for continued contributions and continual improvement.

Education and training

In industry, "training" is a more common term than "education." With a training mind-set, managers can come across as demanding a certain activity because the regulation "says so" rather than because "it's the best way to do it."

Leaders educate — offering rationale and examples rather than policy and directives. This enables individuals or teams to customize patient-safety procedures that best fit their situation. This process of refining a set of procedures allows people to assume ownership and follow through from a self-directed or responsible perspective.[1]

Communication

Under pressure to get a job done, managers often speak first and listen later. This is a reasonable strategy for efficient action. After describing an action plan

Expert Q&A   Getting "buy-in"

David Page is president and chief executive officer of Fairview Health Services, Minneapolis, Minnesota, and chair of Safest in America, a coalition of ten healthcare systems and 27 hospitals in the Minneapolis-St. Paul area plus the Mayo Clinic in Rochester, Minnesota.

Q   *You sit at the top of a very large organization — seven hospitals, 31 primary-care clinics, 28 specialty clinics, 18,900 employees. Your annual report displays photos of various employees, each with the caption, "I am Fairview." As CEO, what are you doing to get thousands of employees to internalize that belief?*

A   *Well, we have an awfully good head start in getting visceral buy-in since most people in healthcare come with some sense of calling for service. I don't want to disparage anyone, but our jobs aren't selling insurance or cars or shoes at the mall.*

Where that belief — "I am Fairview" — really manifests itself is in the exchange between caregivers and patients and their families. I'm a good distance from that exchange. My job is to hold up those people who manifest the belief.

There is absolutely no way I can spend enough time doing the things that need to be done for safety. Forty, fifty hours a week is not enough. But a significant part of what any CEO does is symbolic. People look at the CEO and make interpretations all the time. I know I should model all the time. I must model the belief and connect and link it to our employees throughout our organization.

Our mission is manifested through touching, when we touch patients and their families. Now if you're in accounting or the motor pool, you might feel you're not part of the mission. I've got to let those people know they are all part of it, whether it's a security guard on the third shift in the behavioral unit or a neurosurgeon in OR. They are all part of the same team.

It's like the story about the janitor at NASA. When he's asked what his job is, he says it's sending a rocket to the moon.

We need our people to be proud of being part of a quality organization. When I go out on these "gee-whiz, how-do-you-do-that?" walkarounds, I might watch a nurse in the neonatal ICU handling a tiny, tiny baby with a cracked chest after surgery. And I'll say, "My god, I want to be part of that organization." That's the feeling I want everyone to have.

Case study A CEO's currency: time and attention

Brock Nelson is the president and chief executive officer of Regions Hospital in St. Paul, Minnesota.

Q *Every single day of 2003, your hospital averaged 166 emergency center visits, 29 surgery center cases and 657 outpatient visits. How can there not be slips, mistakes, oversights and miscommunication, given this high level of patient-care activity?*

A *You're right. The number of opportunities for bad exchanges and missed hand-offs, for example, is immense. But that's not an excuse. You just do not accept the response, "It can't be fixed."*

Clearly this sets the stage for the need for patient-safety work. There are a variety of mechanisms to embed the values and practices of our Patient's Bill of Rights. Transparency is very important. We require direct conversations with patients about errors. We expect these conversations to be held.

The biggest principle is no one should fear retaliation for disclosing error. My own experience with disclosure is you reduce malpractice claims the more transparent you are. It is a myth to think hiding errors will reduce claims.

We survey every patient and we've learned safety is an increased priority with them, clearly a growing concern. But their responses or reac-

and accountability system, managers then field questions from workers who want to make sure they will do the right thing.

Leaders take time to learn another person's perspective before offering direction, advice, or support. "Executive walkarounds" is a practice gaining currency in patient safety. Active listening is key to any walkaround, to diagnosing a situation. To be sure, this is not the most efficient approach to getting a job done. It requires patience and a communication approach that asks many questions before delivering advice — which is why it can be a struggle getting execs engaged in floor-level patient-safety activities. But this is indeed how leaders bring values to life, and how they help individuals or teams troubleshoot and problem-solve.

Motivation

Managers seek efficiency. Compliant behavior, following prescribed requirements, is efficient. But behaviors performed to comply with an accreditation goal or system directive are accomplished to satisfy someone else — and they are likely to cease or slacken when they cannot be monitored.

Leaders present a reasonable rationale for a desired outcome — why patient-safety performance must improve — and then offer opportunities for *tions didn't overwhelm us. You're not opening Pandora's Box by surveying patients. By asking for feedback from them or their representatives, you're obviously listening. Then we play back to patients what we think we've heard. This is important because we have a very diverse group of patients, with diverse languages and cultures.*

New employee orientations are another mechanism to embed safety. I do them myself if I'm available. Time and attention is said to be the currency of CEOs. That's the most important thing I can offer patient safety. Patient safety applies to everyone, all of our more than 3,000 employees. A parking-lot attendant, for example, has a duty to act if he sees a suspicious person. The outcome could be harm, or making a person feel unsafe.

Everyone has a role in safety. It could be in the pharmacy, in the food service, with student interns in the lab double-checking labels to make sure they match. In that case, it's not just matching numbers, it's making sure Mrs. Smith's tissue matches up, because it could be life or death right there.

You also need to staff for safety. We have a specific individual assigned as our patient-safety manager. We also participate in national and state patient-safety associations and initiatives.

You need to spread the message of safety at every point in the organization. We have a really good director of communication who routinely issues reports on safety. You need consistency with your safety message, a consistent format, a consistent language.

others to customize methods for achieving that outcome. They facilitate a special kind of motivation that comes from inside people. It is not directed by others. People participate because they want to, not because they have to.

Flexibility

Most behavior on any job starts because someone asked for it. The important issue is whether behavior remains other-directed or advances to self-directed. This depends to some extent on how you ask.

Managers tend not to ask but rather command. But this type of controlled behavior is likely to require constant "management."

Leaders raise expectations rather than issue commands. Expectations imply choice. When people realize what's expected of them but perceive some personal control in how to reach specific goals, they are more likely to own the process and move from depending on the directions of others to directing themselves.

Measurement

Managers focus on the numbers. This brings us to an interesting topic: One of the emerging debates in patient safety centers on the so-called "business case" for justifying investments in reducing risks and protecting patients. Where's the payback?

We can tell you this question has been analyzed backwards and forwards for at least a century in general industry without adequate resolution. Yes, it's important to know how much a patient-safety training process or IT installation will cost, and the projections for how long will it take for the number or errors or adverse events to come down. But attaching dollar figures to such reductions is: 1) a data-mining exercise that usually produces soft estimates; and 2) of questionable value to a Patient-Safety Culture built on trust and altruism.

When Paul O'Neill was CEO of Alcoa, he publicly threatened to fire any accountant who came to him with a cost analysis of accident reductions.[2] O'Neill's vision as a leader was to use his workforce's natural compassion for the safety of others to bind together Alcoa's culture of commitment and collaboration. If employees saw safety equated to profit and loss, it became a cold management priority — not an organic cultural value.

Leaders certainly appreciate the need to hold people accountable with numbers — O'Neill loved to talk about Alcoa's impressive declines in injury and illness rates[3] — but leaders also understand you can't measure everything. There are issues like patient safety where you raise expectations of performance because it's the responsible and humane thing to do — to do no harm. In the process, leaders such as O'Neill perceive opportunities to increase self-esteem, self-efficacy, personal control, optimism, and a sense of belonging throughout a culture. And there are hard-to-quantify competitive advantages — being seen as "best in class" or world class, an enhanced reputation in the marketplace, and positive relations with stakeholders (community leaders, customers/patients, the media, lawmakers, state and federal agencies, etc.)

The bottom line (and we hesitate to use this term in light of what we've just said): safety management represents oversight at an operations level needed to meet predetermined requirements. But a Patient-Safety Culture is built on more than meeting requirements. Patient-safety specialists know when to manage, and when to lead, when to hold people accountable, and when to build responsibility.

Managers vs. Leaders

Managers...
- *Go by the numbers*
- *Emphasize training*
- *Speak first, then listen*
- *Strive for compliance*
- *Lean on mandates*
- *Live by measurements.*

Leaders...
- *Focus on activities*
- *Emphasize education*
- *Listen first, then speak*
- *Offer opportunities*
- *Emphasize expectations*
- *Don't measure everything.*

2 Trust

Create a secure and protective environment for fledgling safety cultures

Trust is like a steel cable wrapped many times around this fragile thing called culture, creating a secure and protective environment. So how can we increase levels of trust within a system to improve patient safety? The following words — all beginning with the letter "C" — capture the essence of trust-building. Use them to kick off your own discussion of trust within a team or unit.

Communication

There is probably no better way to earn someone's trust in your intentions regarding patient safety, your plans and goals, than by listening attentively to what that person has to say. It's active listening, as we've described earlier. Listen to others first before laying out your agenda, and you increase the chance they will reciprocate and listen to you. Plus, you also learn how to present your message to get the best possible understanding, appreciation, and agreement.

Caring

When you take the time to listen, you send a most important message that you care. And when people believe you care about them, they will care about what you tell them.

Asking questions also communicates caring and builds trust. Not typically bland questions like, "How are you doing?" but deeper, more penetrating questions. Questions targeting a specific aspect of a person's job send the signal you care about him or her. You're showing genuine interest in what people are doing and how they feel.

A staff person of one CEO we interviewed commented, without any prompting: "He is the kind of leader who knows me, my name, about my family and what's new in my life. That's because he asks and then, God bless him, remembers what I said."

Candor

We trust people who are frank and open with us, without being tactless. They get right to the point, whether setting an expectation for patient safety or giving feedback. As Collins stresses in his bestselling book, *Good to Great*, leaders of world-class organizations communicate the brutal facts to everyone involved.[4] Then problem-solving communications can be people-based.

"Sometimes you have to rain on parades," one CEO of a healthcare system told us, recalling a time when he saw room for improvement in hospital-acquired infection rates while "the troops" were celebrating progress. At a safety meeting, he balanced his appreciation for the progress that had been made with raising the fact a patient had just recently suffered an adverse event relating to infection.

Candor also requires a lack of prejudice. Candid people are not judgmental.

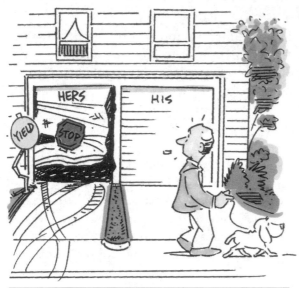

We all tend not to trust people who show a tendency to evaluate or judge others on the basis of some stereotype or preconceived notion. How fair is that person going to be? Even when their prejudice is not directed toward you, are you going to trust their abilities and intentions?

Consistency

We usually trust the intentions of people who confess openly their inability to answer our question. But we expect them to follow through when they say they'll get back

Stereotyping is mindless and unfair.

to us. What happens when they don't — when their actions are not consistent with their words?

Whether the promise regards a positive reward or negative threat of punishment, trust decreases when the consequence is not delivered.

Commitment

People who are dependable and reliable are not only consistent, they demonstrate commitment. This is critical when it comes to safety-related issues. Safety lends itself to warm motherhood-and-apple pie speeches, but not always hard follow-up financial investments. From years of observing safety practices in general industry, we can tell you employees possess a built-in skepticism when it comes to management safety pledges.

Consensus

When a group of people reach consensus about something, group members signal trust in the opinions or recommendations of others. If a decision is reached that leaves out a minority view, there might be active or passive resistance on the part of those who have been "lost" in the process. Without everyone's buy-in, commitment, and involvement, we can't trust the process to come off as expected.

So how do you develop group consensus? It requires candid, consistent, caring communication among all members of a discussion or decision-making group. In her book, *Teamwork from Start to Finish*,[5] Fran Rees lists six basic steps to reach a consensus decision:

• Decide the aim or purpose of the consensus-building exercise.

• Spell out the criteria needed to make the group decision acceptable. One criterion might be to stay within budget constraints.

• Gather information useful for making the decision.

• Brainstorm possible options; make sure everyone has a chance to voice a personal opinion.

• Evaluate options against the group's criteria. Which solutions meet the "must have" criteria? Which options meet the "nice but not necessary" criteria? Can certain options be combined to meet both criteria?

• Make the final decision as a team. Which option or combination of options best meets all of the "necessary" criteria and most of the "desirable" criteria? Who has reservations and why? How can individual skepticism be resolved? Can everyone support the most popular option? What can be altered in the most popular action plan to attract unanimous support and ownership? We're sure you see there's no quick fix to reaching consensus.

Character

All of the characteristics of a trusting culture are practiced by a person of character. Admitting vulnerability and the need for feedback is also a sign of character. "I didn't contribute much to that meeting," recalled a hospital executive who convened an emergency meeting in his office the morning after learning of a patient's death due to a preventable mistake. But he needed to hear what his staff had to say.

③ Embedding

Integrate safety into everyday ACTS: acting, coaching, thinking and seeing

How do you get ready for work in the morning? After getting out of bed we usually follow a regular routine before leaving the house. Many of these "get-ready" behaviors are considered priorities — important, but not always essential.

Now imagine getting up late. Do you shift your priorities? You might skip your stretching or exercise routine, a shower, or even breakfast. But one set of behaviors will never be compromised, because they reflect a value rather than a priority. Yes, we're talking about getting dressed. As young children we are taught to always "cover up" before going out. It's a cultural value, an expectation.

Value-based behaviors are not "add-ons," "afterthoughts" or even part of a "proactive program." Rather, they are activities integrated naturally into a task and deemed indispensable for effectiveness. In a word, these behaviors become "embedded."

In a Patient-Safety Culture, safety must be embedded into the fabric of everyday acting, coaching, thinking and seeing — our ACTS model. More formal practices we've discussed must be similarly embedded:
  • Reporting and analyzing incidents and disseminating finding.
  • Ensuring patient identity
  • Standardizing hand-offs
  • Reconciling medications
  • Ensuring safe use of medications
  • Authentic patient engagement
  • Following CDC hand-hygiene guidelines
  • Conducting risk assessments
  • Ongoing candid and non-punitive conversations about patient issues.
Long after requirements for various patient-safety goals are retired, the

Case Study   *Embedding safety: accept no exceptions*

A registered nurse who is senior director for patient safety describes her organization's attempts at embedding safety into everyday practices.[6]

Q *How do you execute successful patient-safety interventions in the face of time pressures, ongoing distractions, high patient through-put, and unpredictable crises?*

A *Early on we tried some communication and teamwork collaborations around hand-offs that did not get well embedded. Then the new JCAHO goals came along and reignited our efforts. (2006 Critical Access Hospital and Hospital National Patient Safety Goals include implementing a standardized approach to hand-off communications, including an opportunity to ask and respond to questions.)*

One of the first things we did was to get staff in units comfortable with just talking about safety. Briefings and debriefings are important.

It's also important to work in terms of microsystems. Work at the unit level to create microcosms of culture. Allow the unit staff to self-diagnose and set patient-safety priorities.

We've always had an adverse/sentinel event review committee, but we had to get good at getting the learning stories out — what to do differently to be safe.

One of the things we're doing is branding patient-safety communications, using an icon. People are bombarded with information and the staff needs to recognize patient-safety information on bulletin boards.

There is a cultural assessment piece to this, too. We conduct assessments annu-

practices must remain ingrained in daily activity.

But patient-safety measures can indeed come off as "add-ons" — another "job" pushed onto an already full plate. How do we get these responsibilities embedded into the flow of already busy work schedules?

Let's look at how we adjust to new responsibilities in our lives, in a general sense. Most people experience the excitement of developing a new personal relationship. Some of these are considered critical additions to one's life — a gift that adds substantial happiness and a sense of personal fulfillment. You adjust your daily routine to make this new relationship a priority in your life. But we don't always make a relationship integral.

Many circumstances can get in the way:
- distance and time constraints
- previous and current relationships
- communication barriers.

Often family relationships are not integral, leading to conflict, turmoil, and disparaging separations. Some children are viewed as an addition to a family, rather than an integral component, for example. Babysitters are hired,

ally. This is a tool to learn where your patient-safety barriers are, your weak spots that need work. For example, you might learn the hierarchy of the organization can be a barrier to communication openness, to how comfortable people feel to speak up when something's not right.

Embedding safety into your organization takes the support of your leadership, and getting the stories out. People who did the right thing in reporting an event or catching a mistake before it harmed a patient need to know they are backed up. They should be receiving public recognition. These positives reinforce a person's judgment, their decision to act, and help them break through the wall of silence.

The red rules concept is another way to embed safety. Red rules help with situational awareness. A nurse might have five or six patients under her care and can't remember all the procedural nuances. Plus, fatigue can be huge factor. So structured tools — black and white rules — help you check your current mental and behavioral status.

You just called a code. Are you ready to work? What do you have to do? Red rules make certain behaviors and decisions mandatory priorities. They will vary according to department, using the microsystem concept. In OR, one rule for us is before the first scalpel is passed, everyone has to stop and repeat the name of the patient and the procedure.

There must be accountability, discipline, if red rules are violated. No exceptions. Then these stories get out across the organizational lifelines, informal communication lines. That's how organizations "learn," and how practices become reinforced and embedded.

day-care deliveries made, and meal times adjusted to handle an extra mouth to feed. Some quality time might be spent with children, but what are the parents' perceptions?

Do they look forward to and plan for their limited quality time with children (and with each other)? Or, is their day so occupied with job requirements that time with family is unanticipated and merely an "add-on" to a busy day?

Interpersonal relationships improve and persevere to the extent they become embedded in your everyday ACTS — your actions and conversations. Yes relationships call for a certain kind of coaching as well as thinking and seeing (your perceptions). Once embedded, opportunities for interpersonal communication, comfort, and intimacy are perceived as integral — more than an extra "gift" or "positive reinforcer." Your thoughts, fantasies, and even communication with others support and envision opportunities to build and enjoy a relationship. This happens in spite of a hectic schedule that limits occasions for relationship-building and one-on-one appreciation.

Relevance to patient safety

Let's apply this discussion to patient safety. In a robust Patient-Safety Culture, error prevention and guarding patients from harm is incorporated in every aspect of a staff person's work schedule. When patient safety is truly a value, it is not another job or one more headache.

Making patient safety a value is as challenging as cultivating the best kind of relationship. It's far from easy. We've seen many, many organizations in industry struggle mightily trying to embed job safety as a core value. But the more you procrastinate in making relevant behaviors integral — to patient safety or to relationships — the more difficult it can be to achieve the best outcomes. Some delays simply deepen staff resistance or solidify institutional inertia — barriers that become extremely formidable to overcome.

Matter of balance

It's not unusual for personal relationships to be out of balance. One person contributes more than the other. Why? One views the relationship as "integral" while the other considers it an "add-on." This imbalance often fosters emotional upheaval, and frequently ends with someone getting hurt.

Can you see the connection to patient safety? How often do patient-safety coaches, officers and other advocates experience this imbalance when striving to reduce the possibility of errors and failures that harm patients?

Again, we've witnessed in industry how matters of safety are often perceived as an interpersonal confrontation: one person considers safety as integral to the job, the other views it as unnecessary. In healthcare as in industry, many of those who act as if safety is only an extra requirement get lucky and dodge an adverse event, but not everyone. Some do harm because they don't perceive safety as a value integral to their definition of competency.

We hope you'll use life experiences to teach the concept of "embedding" and illustrate its critical role in making patient safety a value. If genuine, relationship examples will surely portray how challenging it is to reach this level of commitment. But your example can also show how rewarding it can be.

4 Selling

Aggressively market patient safety as a "product" with value

Another lesson we've learned over the years from general industry is this: many individuals who take on safety responsibilities — often with intense passion and commitment, we might add — view themselves primarily as subject-matter experts. But certainly not salespeople. In fact, some of these folks cringe at the idea that safety is something that must be sold. "Don't people get it?" they'll complain. They don't want to cheapen safety by marketing it. Apparently salespeople have no place on the moral high ground.

But for patient safety to reach the tipping point in a culture (recall the example in Chapter 1) and then be "tipped" to where it's embedded in your culture, you're going to have to do some selling.

Create positive impressions

Look at it this way: both Madison Avenue ad execs and patient-safety leaders are after a share of mind and loyalty. For both, having their product "out of sight, out of mind" is the kiss of death.

Yes, go ahead and think of patient safety as a "product" — not just a set of rules and policies. And think of doctors, nurses, lab techs and transporters and administrators as your "customers." You want to create an appetite for your product, and get that share of mind. Daily bombardment from competing messages doesn't help matters. So how do you achieve top-of-mind awareness?

How about creating a positive "impression" of patient safety? In advertising the rule is, the more impressions, the more they remember you. It takes at least 12 impressions (messages, signs, personal contacts, emails, etc.) to close a sale, according to Sales and Marketing Management.[7] Most people attempting to make an impression give up after the fourth try.[8] How's your stamina?

"Think about the efforts to get people to stop smoking or start using safety belts," says Jeff Cooper, director of biomedical engineering for Partners HealthCare System, Inc. "The biggest thing is marketing, relentless messaging. It's a practical, relentless pursuit of safety."

Expert Q&A *Pitching patient safety*

A patient-safety advocate who has spent more than a decade engaged in projects to improve the quality of patient care shares her philosophy of "pitching" patient safety.[7]

Q *Over the years, how have you "sold" your patient-safety projects to sponsors and institutions?*

A *We have to show how patient-safety interventions help patients. How they save lives.*

Healthcare fundamentally is about relationships — patient to doctor, doctor to doctor, department to department, doctor to nurse. Forget the systems language nonsense. That's a turn off. We must be very careful with the language we use. Make it relevant to patient care. Show examples of how patient-safety interventions help patients, help doctors and nurses, and strengthen these relationships.

Patient safety is not being pitched right. It's like selling a product. We need to appeal to where people live, to the heart of their real experience. Patient safety should be pitched in terms of solving problems, allowing people to get back to why they went into medicine in the first place.

Research your audience

Marketing safety, like marketing everything from cars, churches, movies and hospitals, should start with market research. How much do you know about your "customers" — your organization's workforce?

Chances are, "consumers" of your patient-safety products share many attributes with the general buying public these days. Healthcare workers are likely to be:

• Skeptical — Fifty-one percent of U.S. workers believe their companies try too hard to "spin" the truth, according to a survey of more than 1,000 "typical" employees.[10]

• Cautious — Employees are not quick to commit. Seventy-three percent of U.S. workers either are not engaged in their work or actively disengaged, according to Gallup.[11]

• Jaded — Two out of every three workers do not identify with or feel motivated to drive their employer's business goals and objectives, according to a survey of 5,000 U.S. households. Less than one-third of all supervisors and managers are perceived to be strong leaders. And only 30 percent of workers claim to be satisfied with educational and training programs.[12] Perhaps too much lip service, too many quick-fix programs, too many slackards held unaccountable. Maybe this is why only half of U.S. workers were happy with their jobs in 2005, down from 59 percent in 1995, according to The Conference Board.[13]

• Confused — Only 51 percent of employees believe their company generally tells employees the truth, according to the survey of "typical" workers. Almost half (48 percent) say they receive more credible information from their direct supervisor than from their company's CEO.[14] Add up these communication gaps and lapses and you have a recipe for confusion.

This could well be the "marketplace" of moods, attitudes and beliefs you're wading into with your patient-safety messages. How do you connect with your target audience and make your message both believable and memorable — one that sticks at the top of people's minds?

Reach customers early

First, you need to reach your "customers" early in their decision-making process — whether or not they're going to buy what you're selling, a package of protocols and procedures called patient safety.

When do employees in your system first form an opinion or make a decision about patient safety — your product?

It could be the first time they walk the floors and notice how clean, or unkempt, your facility is. Housekeeping sends a clear signal about patient care.

Or it might be the quality of their new hire orientation. Is it rushed along with little feeling or enthusiasm? How much time is given to patient safety? At Regions Hospital in St. Paul, Minnesota, CEO Brock Nelson personally conducts these sessions whenever possible. "New employee orientations are another mechanism to embed safety," he told us. "I do them myself if I'm available. Time and attention is said to be the currency of CEOs, that's the most important thing I can offer patient safety."

The quality of early conversations about patient safety will be important. According to internet marketing consultant Willie Crawford,[15] any marketer trying to make a connection and make their message stick should:

• Show you understand what's on your customer's mind. His or her problems, needs, issues. In other words, get out on the floor and start talking. Or more precisely, start probing. Recall from Chapter 1 — ask sincere questions, and really listen. In general industry, we can tell you there is a history of safety officers who venture out of their office only to put out fires and conduct investigations.

• Show you're on their frequency. Remember radio station WIIFM — "what's in it for me" — that we all tune in to (Chapter 1). Patient safety, as passionate as you might feel about it, is not about you, it's about protecting patients. Tap into your employees' own passion for protecting and healing patients. Use "you" and "your" more than "me" and "my" in your communications, both written and verbal.

• Show you have your customers' best interests in mind. Don't be a hero or a know-it-all. You're an advisor, a resource, an honest-broker, a fact-finder, and yes, when needed, an enforcer.

Learn from human nature

Other than Dr. Geller and his researchers at Virginia Tech, no one studies human nature more than advertisers. Here's some of what they've learned that you can use to market patient safety:

People are not impressed by receiving the same message again and again. Patient-safety meetings and training sessions with nothing new to say are sure ways to lose the share-of-mind battle. Recycle old compliance topics and horror stories and watch patient-safety drop out of sight, out of mind.

This calls for aggressive marketing.

• Walk around the floors and make "personal calls," those one-on-one patient-safety contacts.

• Use your hospital web site, annual report, newsletters and email to present patient-safety communications. Arrange a meeting around the growing number of live patient-safety phone-in or desktop seminars.

• Bring in outside speakers for another perspective. Patients or their next-of-kin who experienced harm, or nearly so, can be powerful presenters.

• Customize and personalize patient-safety training content and communications whenever possible.

• Search the internet for interesting, bizarre and informative patient-safety news, statistics and research from around the world. Use search words such as "rapid response teams," "crew resource management," "Patient-Safety Culture," and of course "JCAHO."

• Advertisers have learned that repetition, persistence, and variety — mixing up your messages — matter. Many people aren't in the mood for whatever it is that's being sold when they first hear the message. You want to create what marketing consultant Mark Abraham calls a "dripping tap of information" to reinforce your message.[16]

• When it comes to brand awareness, you want your customers to think of patient safety not just as accreditation goals and requirements — but a necessary part of their job that is caring, creative, responsible, positive, serious and significant.

So how do you do all this without making yourself a pest for patient safety?

Like skilled salespeople, use tact and a sense of timing. Know when to make contact and converse with someone out on the floor and when to pull back. Know when to cut a lecture short. Learn how to edit yourself, sometimes a challenge for knowledge-filled subject matter experts. Again, present yourself as someone who is there to help, to provide answers and info, to educate, not browbeat into submission and compliance.

Expert Q&A *Relentless messaging*

Jeffrey B. Cooper, PhD, is a patient safety pioneer. His 1978 paper, "Preventable Anesthesia Mishaps: A study in human factors," was the first in-depth, scientific look at errors in medicine, based on analysis of 359 errors. Today, Dr. Cooper is director of biomedical engineering for Partners HealthCare System, Inc.; associate professor of anesthesia at Harvard Medical School; and executive director of the Center for Medical Simulation in Cambridge, Massachusetts.

Q *In the absence of hard evidence, what will it take to convince the medical community of the efficacy of patient-safety interventions?*

A *It's marketing, PR, organizational communications. Think about the efforts to get people to stop smoking or start using safety belts. The biggest thing is marketing, relentless messaging. It's a practical, relentless pursuit of safety.*

You've got to get people where they live. I tell personal stories of my mistakes, show my vulnerabilities. But you must be careful, because some will see you as weak. You've got to balance being macho, for lack of a better word, with being vulnerable. You modulate your tone. It varies with the audience I'm talking to. Sometimes I need to stand and act more macho because if I come off too touchy-feely the audience will tune me out.

What's been largely missing, but is happening now more, is to use patients' stories. I brought three patients and-or their families to a foundation's board retreat to tell their stories, and the response was far more than I anticipated. Two stories related to overt errors. In one, a husband died. In another, a son was left paralyzed. People at the meeting were blown away. These stories are powerful.

⑤ Empathy

Know when to coach, instruct, support or delegate

When it comes to patient safety, your culture needs your leadership. More importantly, it needs the right kind of leadership. After all, you can insult people with too much direction, or confuse them with too little. To effectively take the lead in reducing error and protecting patients, you need to know what style of leadership is required. This means practicing empathic observing, listening, and questioning.

As discussed in Chapter 3 – Coaching, we are empathic when we put ourselves in the other person's shoes before diagnosing a behavior-related problem and offering advice for improvement.

Let's consider four different ways you can lead others. At any point in time you can coach, instruct, support, or delegate, depending on your empathic diagnosis of the situation.[17] To understand the difference between these approaches, recall the basic Activator-Behavior-Consequence paradigm of behavior-based safety detailed in Chapter 2 – Acting. "A" stands for activator or the various conditions or events that precede behavior ("B") and direct it. "C" refers to the consequences that follow behavior and influence whether it will occur again. Consequences motivate behavior.

Coaching

Coaches give direction and provide feedback. They present a plan, perhaps specific behaviors needed for a certain task, and then follow-up with support and empathic correction to pinpoint what worked and what did not. Periodic activators (direction) keep people on the right track, while intermittent consequences (feedback) provide motivation to keep people going.

The change process

Introducing patient-safety values and activities is a change process. It's worth noting these five levels of participation in a change process:

- *leaders or innovators who are totally involved;*
- *those who want to participate but need a little direction and support;*
- *those (usually the majority) who are neutral or nervous about change and need prodding and encouragement from others;*
- *passive resisters who are critical and untrusting of something new imposed on them, and use apathy and cynicism as excuses to remain uninvolved; and*
- *active resisters who view change as a threat or a loss of personal control, and might exert measures (especially if they are in positions of authority) to stifle the participation of others.*

Active resisters stick out and attract attention. Non-participants use them to rationalize their own commitment to stay in their comfort zones. Managers aim their attention on these individuals, sometimes using punitive measures. But this only builds resentment of the system among all resisters, and makes it less likely they'll join your change process.

Instead, focus your early momentum-building efforts on participants rather than nonparticipants.

Delegating

Sometimes it's best to give an assignment in general terms (without specific directions) and to limit interpersonal behavior-focused feedback. This is true when team members are already motivated to do their best and will give each other direction, support, and feedback when needed. These individuals should be self-accountable (or responsible), and expected to use self-management techniques (activators and consequences) to keep themselves motivated and on the right track.

Instructing

Some people are already highly motivated to perform well, but don't know exactly what to do. This is often the case with new hires, temps or transfers. In this case, you need to focus on giving behavior-focused instruction.

Supporting

What about the experienced nurse or doctor who does the same tasks day after day? This individual doesn't need your direction, but could benefit if you periodically give sincere thanks for a job well done.

Watch for those who display immediate interest and commitment to patient safety. These individuals are innovators who have dramatic positive influence on the rest of the staff. Encourage those totally involved in the process (Level 1) to help people who believe in the change but are not yet totally immersed (Level 2). Then these two groups can work with the majority (Level 3) who need direction, support, and examples to follow.

Be aware of the need to develop feelings of competence among potential participants. Many might like your new plan but are unsure of their ability to handle the change. Give these folks all the education and skills training they need.

What about the resisters? Leave them alone — unless their actions pose risks to patients that demand immediate intervention. Don't give them opportunities (through punishment, for example) to dig in and become more committed to their contrary opinions. Give them opportunities to receive training and participate in the new process when they decide it's worth their effort. That will happen soon after the majority of the workforce recognizes the change is beneficial and gets involved in continuous improvement.

When the change becomes the norm, the passive resisters (Level 4) will feel the peer pressure and fall in line. Some active resisters (Level 5) may never engage beyond superficial rules compliance. Monitoring and disciplinary action may be necessary to ensure their actions remain harmless to patients.

Competence and commitment

So how do you know which leadership style to use? This is where empathy comes into play. Size up situations and people — through observing, listening, and questioning — to determine what approach to use. Look for two critical characteristics: competence and commitment.

Coaching is needed when a person's competence and commitment regarding your patient-safety activities are relatively low. You can improve competence through specific direction and feedback, and increase commitment by sincerely giving appreciation and support. Anything that increases a person's perception of importance or self-worth on the job can enhance commitment. What makes that happen? It's not always obvious, but if you listen, observe, and ask questions you'll find out.

Delegating is relevant when people know what to do (competence) and are motivated to do it (commitment). Delegating leaders provide clear expectations and show sincere appreciation for worthwhile work. They enable self-direction and self-motivation.

Empathic leaders usually know when an individual or patient-safety team advances to this level because they have observed successive progress. But it's often useful to ask people whether they are ready for this style of leadership. If they say "no," then ask what they need to reach this stage. Do they need more competence through direction? More commitment through some kind of support the organization could make available?

Supportive leadership is needed when people know what to do for patient safety, but don't always follow through. This problem can't be solved with direction or training, and it can be a cause of great concern and frustration. Low motivation and commitment to patient safety can cause grievous harm, so you must show support for the values of the culture as well as empathy (a sense of justice) for the individuals.

Instructive leadership is called for when people are internally motivated to perform well, but don't know how to maximize their efforts. In this case, empathic leaders focus on giving specific behavior-based directions. The figure here shows these four

Competence

	Low	High
Low	*Coaching*	*Supporting*
High	*Instructing*	*Delegating*

(vertical axis label) **Commitment**

Leadership style is determined by the level of competence and commitment.

types of leadership styles as they are influenced by the recipient's level of competence and commitment.

Don't keep it a secret

Empathic leadership works best when everyone involved understands the four approaches and the two critical factors that determine the need for one style over others. Then people can request a certain leadership style from their flexible and empathic leaders.

You might want to consider the benefits of telling people what leadership style you plan to use, asking permission for a particular approach, or asking an individual or team what style they would prefer. This is particularly useful when moving from one approach to another. If you feel it's time to move from giving instructions to delegating, announce your change and explain the reasons.

Flex leaders

Leadership styles change depending on circumstances. Whether you coach, instruct, support, or delegate depends on your periodic assessments of what's needed. Since people and organizations are dynamic and always changing, so will your leadership styles.

The new employee needs patient-safety instruction at first, for example. As he or she becomes familiar with routines, your support will be more important than instruction. If you later decide to expand the person's patient-safety responsibilities, you'll probably need to be a coach, providing both direction and support, at least at first. Eventually, a delegating approach might be most appropriate. The employee is now self-directed and self-motivated. Remember to give genuine words of appreciation when your expectations are met.

6 Momentum

Leverage achievement, atmosphere and attitude

How can you harness momentum to improve your patient-safety processes?

Coaches are very aware of the power of momentum. For example, research published in the *Journal of Applied Behavior Analysis* in 1991 systematically analyzed 14 college basketball games during the 1989 NCAA tournament and found that basketball coaches called time-out from play when being outscored by their opponents an average of 2.63 to 1.0.[18] Calling time-out usually stopped the other team's momentum — the rate of successful plays during the three minutes immediately after a time-out was nearly equal for both teams.

Let's consider factors relevant to accelerating momentum. In interviews for this book we talked with several healthcare leaders who expressed frustration at the slow pace of getting patient-safety-related behaviors and practices adopted in their cultures. We can return to the sports analogy for intuitive answers to the question, "How do we build and maintain momentum?" We think you'll agree from personal experience that three factors are critical to momentum-building:

- Achievement of the team
- Atmosphere of the culture
- Attitude of the leaders.

The three ingredients start with the letter "A," so they're easy to remember. And notice that they are clearly overlapping and interrelated.

Achievement

It's obvious that success builds success. Good performance is more likely after you're on a "roll" of successful behaviors than failures. In sports, a succession of gains or winning plays or points creates momentum.

Sports psychologists talk about momentum as a gain in psychological power — including confidence, self-efficacy, and personal control — that changes perceptions and attitudes, and enhances both mental and physical performance. It all starts with noticing a run of individual or team achievements. So how do you get on a roll with patient-safety initiatives?

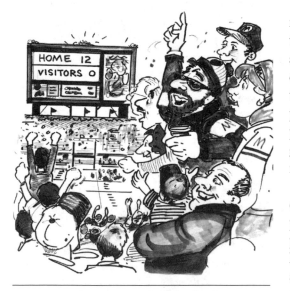

A winning score builds momentum.

You've got to keep score. You need a system to track small wins that can build momentum. At sporting events, fans constantly check the scoreboard to measure their team's performance. This is a prime reason we like to watch or participate in sporting events. We get objective and fair feedback regarding ongoing performance.

"Knowing the score" creates excitement if our team is performing well, or urgency if performance must improve. This kind of observable and equitable appraisal is a performance measure that can be used as feedback to improve subsequent performance and increase the probability of more success and continued momentum.

To successfully embed patient safety into an organizational culture, we must find an ongoing objective and impartial measure of performance that allows us to regularly evaluate our progress. When employees see continuous improvement in their patient- safety "score," they recognize momentum and stay motivated to participate in the achievement-oriented process.

This is why in People-Based Patient Safety we emphasize the need to:

• Develop up-stream process measures (such as number of audits completed or percentage of safe behaviors);

• Set process-oriented goals that are SMART—specific, motivational, achievable, relevant, trackable, and shared;

• Discuss performance in terms of achievement — what people have done for patients, and what additional achievement potential is within their domain of control;

• Recognize individuals appropriately for their accomplishments; and

• Celebrate group or team accomplishments on a regular basis.

Expert Q&A *"Significant improvement is possible"*

Rosemary Gibson is the author of *Wall of Silence*, published in 2003, and senior program officer at the Robert Wood Johnson Foundation, where she works on the foundation's initiatives to improve quality of patient care.

Q *In the broad sense, how much patient-safety improvement is realistic, given the nursing shortage, the long hours put in by physicians, and the aging Baby Boomer population putting more demands and stresses on the healthcare system?*

A *Significant improvement in patient safety is possible.*

As an example, rapid response teams are a patient-safety intervention that hospitals are implementing to reduce deaths from failure to rescue. The teams respond to calls from nurses and others when a patient exhibits deteriorating clinical signs and symptoms. Responding usually within five minutes, the teams assess and treat patients as necessary.

Hospitals have experienced reductions in codes of up to 26 percent. Nurses, especially med-surg nurses, value the back-up system of expertise the teams provide. At least one hospital has used its rapid response team as a tool to recruit nurses, and other hospitals report the teams increase nurse retention.

This intervention demonstrates it is possible to improve patient safety and improve the work environment for nurses and doctors who are taking care of more complex, high-risk patients.

Atmosphere

In sports, it's called the "home-field advantage." It means having your band and your fans on hand to create or sustain momentum. By packing the stands and cheering loudly, fans create an atmosphere that can motivate the home team to try harder. A run of successful plays can lead to a score, and then momentum to achieve more. This stimulates the home crowd to cheer louder, and momentum is supported.

The relevance to patient safety should be clear. The atmosphere surrounding your processes will influence the degree of participation in your activities. Is your culture optimistic about the patient-safety effort, or is the process viewed as another "flavor of the month?" Does staff trust management to give adequate resources to a long-term commitment, or is this a "knee-jerk" reaction to media bashing or accreditation goals or a "me-too" leap on a bandwagon that will soon give way to other emerging issues, crises or priorities?

Before helping a work team implement a People-Based Safety™ process in industry, Dr. Geller's partners at Safety Performance Solutions insist everyone in the organization learn the principles underlying the process. Everyone in the culture needs to learn the rationale behind the safety process, even those who will not be involved in actual implementation. This helps to provide the right kind of atmosphere or cultural context to support momentum.

When the vision of an implementation team is shared optimistically with the entire workforce, people are likely to buy in and do what it takes to support the mission. When this happens, interpersonal trust and morale builds, along with a winning spirit. People don't fear failure but expect to succeed, and this atmosphere fuels more achievement from the process team.

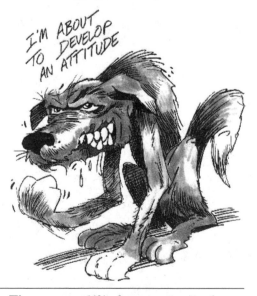

The wrong attitude saps momentum.

Attitude

The coach of an athletic team can make or break momentum. Coaches initiate and support momentum by helping team members and the team as a whole recognize their accomplishments. This starts with a clear statement of a vision and attainable goals. Then the leader enthusiastically holds individuals and the team accountable for achieving these goals.

A positive coach can even help members of a losing team feel better about themselves, and give momentum a chance. The key is to find pockets of excellence to acknowledge, thus building self-confidence and self-efficacy. Then specific corrective feedback will be heard and accepted as key to being more successful and building more momentum.

It does little good for safety leaders to reprimand individuals or teams for a poor safety record, unless they also provide a method people can use to do better. And the leader must explain and support the improvement method with confidence, commitment, and enthusiasm.

This point warrants closer examination: The way patient-safety setbacks or "defeats" are handled within a culture is a critical question. We've learned from industry that safety can be a demoralizing "game" because defeats — accidents, injuries, errors and mistakes — are so much more glaring and obvious than victories. To heap blame and shame on top of the obvious just pushes the team further away from its goals.

In contrast, "victory" in safety means nothing went wrong, no one got hurt. Where's the evidence of victory, one might ask? The outcome is invisible. The patient goes home without complications, as expected. So for momentum to build and continue, you need to search for success stories to recognize and celebrate:

• A rapid response team that successfully saved a crashing patient.

• A transporter who spotted a mislabeled specimen.

• A coach who worked with a long-term care patient to bring dangerously high blood sugar levels under control.

• A team that brought MRSA infections down to practically zero in a post-surgical unit.

• A unit that improved

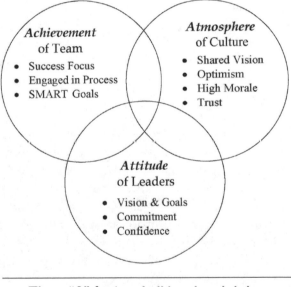

Three "A" factors build and maintain momentum.

hand-hygiene compliance from 50 to 75 percent on its way to a vision of 100 percent.

• A unit that delivered medications on schedule to patients 99 percent of the time for the last three months.

Taking time out of hectic days to recognize these kinds of accomplishments helps develop feelings of achievement among those directly involved (the team) and an optimistic atmosphere from others (the work culture). These are the ingredients for safety momentum. Keep these in place and your momentum will be sustained. Then you can truly expect the best from your efforts to implement People-Based Patient Safety.™

7 Celebration

Focus on your journey, not just your outcomes

Surveys by The Gallup Organization indicate 59 percent of employees are not engaged by their work (effectively checked out and essentially sleepwalking through their jobs, putting time but not energy or passion), and 14 percent are actively disengaged (busy acting out their unhappiness and undermining accomplishments of engaged coworkers).[19] "Lean and mean" downsizing has indeed shaken spirits in many organizations, leading to apathy, helplessness, and less willingness to look out for the safety and health of others, or in healthcare systems, taking extra precautions to prevent harm from reaching patients. Employees in the U.S. feel dissatisfied and disconnected from their employees at an alarmingly high rate.[20] What can we do in response?

Giving and receiving quality recognition, as we just discussed, are prime ways to boost morale. Let's talk about a specific form of recognition: celebrations. When done correctly, patient-safety celebrations can be an antidote for sagging morale. They can motivate teamwork, build a sense of belonging, and boost caregivers' desire to act on their intrinsic desire to watch out for patients. The key is the phrase "when done correctly." Here are guidelines you can follow:

Don't celebrate cheating

It's quite common for companies in industry to hold annual safety dinners or picnics. And this is often the occasion for a "suit" from the front office to step to the microphone and congratulate a department, a shift or perhaps an entire facility for working a particular number of weeks or months with no recordable injury. This kind of achievement is indeed worth celebrating, but let's be sure the record was reached fairly. If people cheat to win — not reporting injuries, for example — the celebration won't mean much.

We like the idea of celebrating the success of process activities. For example, patient-safety-related behaviors needed from employees to warrant a celebration can be specified. A group might decide to celebrate after completing a designated number of audits, investigating a given number of near-hit reports, or completing a certain number of one-on-one safety coaching sessions. In these cases, an achievable goal is set and progress monitored. When the goal is reached, a celebration is clearly earned.

We understand how difficult it is to pull everyone together for a formal celebration in the midst of caring for a unit full of patients, when physicians are often off-site and when other shifts are off-duty. But we know of hospitals that hold annual patient-safety days where everyone is invited, and any recognition of achievements is communicated electronically throughout the system for the benefit of those off-site or who otherwise were not present. Brainstorm on how best to build celebration time into the schedule.

Where there's a reason to celebrate, you'll discover a way.

Focus on the journey

Most safety celebrations we've seen in industry give far too little attention to the journey — the processes that contribute to reaching the milestone. Typically, the focus is on the end result, like achieving zero injuries for a certain period of time. When you pinpoint processes instrumental to reaching a safety milestone, you give valuable direction and motivation. Participants learn what they need to do to continue a successful journey.

Plus, employees who are responsible for the behaviors identified as contributing to the safety outcome receive a special boost. They feel effective, in control, and optimistic. This reinforces their internal "scripts" for later self-motivation.

But perhaps the most important reason for acknowledging journey activities is it gives credit where credit is due. The people and actions that made the difference are endorsed.

Recipients should be participants

As we mentioned, in your typical safety celebration managers give and employees receive — certainly an impressive show of top-down support. But the ceremony would be more memorable and beneficial as a learning and motivational experience if employees played a larger role. Managers should listen more than speak — and they should stick around. We've seen and heard of too many safety celebrations where the boss heads for the exit after making what amounts to a cameo appearance.

Relive the experience

Management's primary role in a safety celebration should be to facilitate discussions of activities that led to success. The best safety celebration Dr. Geller ever observed was planned by employees and featured a series of brief presentations by teams of hourly workers. Numerous safety ideas were shared. Some workers showed off new personal protective equipment, some displayed graphs of data obtained from environmental or behavioral audits, some discussed their procedures for encouraging near-hit reports and implementing corrective action, and one group presented its ergonomic analysis and redesign of a workstation.

Don't ignore failures

Work teams in this celebration discussed both success and failures, displaying positive results and recalling disappointments, dead ends, and frustrations. Pointing out the highs and lows made their presentations realistic, and underscored the amount of dedication needed to complete their projects and contribute to the celebrated reduction in injuries.

You justify a celebration by showing how difficult it was to reach the milestone. Pointing out hardships along the way reflects the fact luck was not involved. Many people went beyond the call of duty to contribute and collaborate.

Make it memorable

One week after the safety celebration described here, each participant received a framed photograph of everyone who attended the event. Tangible rewards reinforce the memory of an occasion and promote its value. Ideally, the memento should have a safety theme or slogan and be something that can be displayed or used at workstations — coffee mugs, for example. In a unit of a children's hospital, small foam wedges of swiss cheese were handed out as "stress relievers" — and reminders of the swiss cheese analogy used to explain how mistakes can occur and patients harmed when a series of errors align like the holes in slices of swiss cheese.

Go one-on-one

In every group, some individuals take charge and champion the effort, while others sit back and "go with the flow." In fact, some people exert less effort when working with a group than when working alone. Behavioral scientists call this phenomenon "social loafing."[18]

When you recognize the champions of a group effort one-on-one, you let them know you realize the importance of their leadership. This adds to the motivation received from the earlier group celebration and increases the likelihood of their continued leadership.

One final thought: everyone has his or her own way of enjoying success. And when it comes to group celebration we often inadvertently impose our prejudices on others. When you ask people how they want to celebrate as a group, challenge them to go beyond tangible rewards. The celebration shouldn't be seen as a payoff. You want a meaningful and memorable event that can serve as a stepping stone for greater achievements.

8 Social influences

Barriers or boosts to your patient-safety initiatives

Here are seven principles gleaned from social science research that can inhibit or facilitate long-term participation in patient-safety activities. We're talking about basic social dynamics that reflect — and influence — the patient-safety culture of a healthcare system. Use these social influence principles to analyze the dynamics that hinder optimal involvement in your activities, and decide which can be changed to fuel more participation.[22]

1) We strive to be consistent

Commitments are most influential when they are public, active, and perceived as voluntary or not coerced. When we make a choice or take a stand, we face personal and social pressures to stick to our commitment. So it's better to have employees make a public rather than a private commitment to perform a certain safe behavior, which can take place at a safety meeting or team meeting.

2) We want to return a favor

Basically, if you're nice to people, they will feel obligated to return the favor. What does this mean for patient safety? "Never leave your wingman," as they say at Sentara Healthcare in Virginia. When you take the time to double check, to verify, or otherwise act to help a coworkers avoid a slip or mistake, you set the tone for what is called "reciprocity." You increase the likelihood a person will actively care for the safety of someone else.

3) We help those we like

Who will you go out of your way to help or care for — someone you like or dislike? It's obvious, right? So we need to build positive relationships in our workplaces. How? Here are three strategies:

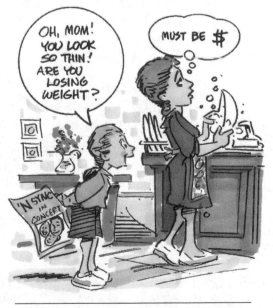

Insincere recognition can feel like behavior modification.

• Emphasize similarities: "Birds of a feather flock together." Through initial informal conversation and astute observation, you can find common bonds between you and others you'd like to influence. Maybe you enjoy the same hobbies or recreational activities. Or maybe you have matching educational backgrounds or employment histories, or have similar opinions about current events, corporate issues, and even politics.

• Give praise: Genuine one-to-one praise, recognition, and rewarding feedback build relationships. The person you reward likes you more; and because their behavior deserves recognition, your appreciation for that person increases.

• Promote cooperation: Cooperation works better than contests and competition in forging positive relationships. You want to build a sense of interdependency toward achieving a common goal. We're more likely to work with, and help, those we depend on.

4) We follow the crowd

We see examples of conformity every day, in the types of clothes people wear, their styles of communication and the products we buy. Don't overlook the power of conformity in influencing participation. The pressure to conform is greater when the consensus (say a commitment to patient safety) comes out of a large group, as well as when group members are seen as relatively experienced.

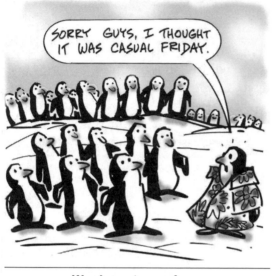

We dress to conform.

People look for guidance in unfamiliar situations — though custom or unwritten rules may prevent them from expressing it. Experienced staff should feel especially responsible to model safe work practices to new hires, floaters, interns and residents, temps and transfers. There are daily opportunities for this in the mentoring system so integral to medical education.

5) We respect authority

Mentors and role models have credible authority. In healthcare's hierarchy they wield significant influence. But there's a flip side to the power of authority. Following orders gives us an excuse to escape taking personal responsibility for what we are doing. If someone with authority tells us to take a risk, we're often willing to comply because if something goes wrong, it won't be our fault. We can blame the person who told us to do it. Be aware of the power of authority, and encourage people to resist the temptation to follow orders blindly and mindlessly.

6) We want what is hard to get

The value of something — front-row seats at a game, Elvis's autograph, new episodes of "The Sopranos," antique furniture — increases with the perception of scarcity. People will collect, go out of their way to purchase, and get caught up in bids and bargains for items considered scarce.

So what can the scarcity principle teach us about getting more people involved in a patient-safety process?

• *Emphasize unique features:* Patient-safety experts are aware of best practices, what other healthcare systems are doing, or not doing. In fact, they are likely the only staff possessing this knowledge. So use it. Show how a particular initiative you're rolling out is leading edge. When people believe they have an opportunity to pilot a new approach to patient safety, their motivation is powered by the scarcity principle.

Of course the flip side here are the skeptics who will look at your pilot project and throw down the challenge: "Show me the data. Where's the evidence this will work?"

To which Jeff Cooper responds: "Sometimes I ask, 'Is there nothing you'll buy on face validity?' What's the ROI on a one-hour lecture for clinicians? Some things in medicine are completely driven by anecdotal evidence. You've got to do some things that reasonable people agree on."

• *Play up the fear of losing:* Social psychologists have shown that people are especially motivated to avoid a loss. Think about it. When it's evident you need to act immediately in order to avoid harming a patient, you are aroused to mindful action.

So how do we demonstrate the harm that can come from unsafe acts and hazardous environments? Personal testimonies from patients harmed due to preventable error, or staff involved in such cases, are powerful reminders of what's at stake. But such participation, by staff in particular, will come only in a so-called non-punitive culture, one where actions (disclosure is appreciated, not denigrated) speak louder than promises.

7) We want what is novel

We are drawn to what is new or different as well as what is scarce or rare. The novelty principle is reflected in our desire for excitement and surprise in our relationships with others. This appeal of newness and unpredictability facilitates the beginning of a relationship, while the lack of novelty in a familiar routine can be the key factor in the breakup of a relationship.

The implication for patient safety? The uniqueness of a new initiative can promote initial curiosity, interest and involvement; but over time, the same routine can seem dull and uninspiring, leading to a drop in the quantity or quality of participation. This is a problem inherent in stringent safety rules that allow little leeway for originality.

It's important to find ways to vary aspects of a particular safety process. Actually, it's essential for continuous improvement. A mechanism for continually refining and upgrading your procedures should be established at the start. This usually requires the ongoing involvement of a patient-safety team or steering committee that solicits and reviews staff suggestions for program refinement, decides which refinement(s) to implement first, and then monitors the impact of certain changes to an injury-prevention process.

Your patient-safety teams, task groups and committees not only support the vision of "never-ending improvement," but also maintain a degree of novelty in the error reduction and patient-protection activities of an organization.

FAQ The price of safety is said to be eternal vigilance, which can be exhausting and annoying. How do you keep everyone fresh and focused on patient safety?

The price of competence, which includes safety, is eternal vigilance. If we want to be the best we can be, we need to be open to feedback from others at any time. This is not an easy state to put ourselves in, because we want to feel independent and in control. But the fact is we need others to help us improve.

A critical way to increase competence in healthcare is to include patients as observers. In other words, through patient perception surveys we can learn how to improve. And with behavioral checklists completed by patients we can not only learn how to improve but be motivated to improve from the perspective of the patients we care for.

This can be seen as exhausting and annoying, but only when we don't understand how valuable this process can be. We're suggesting everyone in the healthcare setting, including patients, play a role in a vigilance process. If done correctly the responsibilities will be shared equitably and no single person will be over-taxed.

Of course, it is essential to respond to the results of perception surveys and observation forms. This requires interpersonal conversation and planning in a dynamic fashion. This is not a boring process, but ever-changing and challenging. A "patient-care professional" wants to continually improve, and will use these feedback mechanisms to do so.

It is also important to use genuine recognition as a way to reward those who do improve. Of course, the most powerful reward is the intrinsic reinforcement from a successful process. Healthcare professionals love to hear recognition from their patients. Involving patients in a vigilant or auditing process should increase genuine recognition from patients. This will naturally keep the process fresh and focused on patient safety.

FAQ *How do you keep score with patient safety? How do you know if you are getting better?*

Although trailing metrics, such as the number of adverse events, is the most common approach to evaluating patient safety, it is clearly inferior to leading indicators that reflect proactive processes to prevent errors that adversely impact patient safety.

While the vision is zero errors, zero infections, goals should be set on process activities needed to successively approximate the vision. We're talking about tracking achievements that prevent possibilities of negative consequences to patients. In other words, any measure of what people do to prevent errors in a healthcare system fits this type of score-keeping for patient safety.

For example, audits can be taken intermittently on a number of factors related to error prevention, including housekeeping, task-specific behaviors, and perceptions. The development of a behavioral checklist is invaluable in training individual and group behaviors.

Even more important are the results from using a behavioral checklist. More specifically, a behavioral checklist provides information regarding the percentage of safe behavior per specific category of behaviors. This shows what behaviors may need specific attention with regard to error reduction. Plus, the appropriate use of a checklist activates and supports interdependent communication and coaching. The process of two people discussing behavior-specific feedback develops a sense of belongingness and trust needed to optimize synergy from teamwork.

As for perceptions, we think patients should be surveyed regularly regarding their perceptions of the caretaking they received. Just as students evaluate Dr. Geller's teaching at the end of every semester, patients should evaluate the caretaking they receive per each treatment.

A recent hospital experience for Dr. Geller revealed a number of improvement opportunities, he recalls, but since no one asked his opinion, important feedback was not shared. If he had the opportunity to share his perceptions, the hospital staff could significantly improve their caretaking for the next patient. Without feedback we cannot improve. It's that simple.

Notes

Chapter 1

1. The number of 7,569 hospitals nationwide was reported by the U.S. Census Bureau, April 29, 2005.

2. Kohn, L., Corrigan, J., & Donaldson, M. (2000). *To err is human: Building a safer health system.* Washington, D.C.: Committee on Quality of Health Care in America, Institute of Medicine, National Academy Press. ("The IOM Report").

3. More than 3,000 U.S. hospitals had joined the Institute for Healthcare Improvement's (*www.ihi.org*) 100,000 Lives Campaign as of January, 2006.

4. Wachter, R. M., & Shojania, K. G. (2004). *Internal bleeding: The truth behind America's terrifying epidemic of medical mistakes.* New York: Rugged Land.

5. Devers, K. J., Pham, H. H., & Liu, G. (2004). What is driving hospitals' patient-safety efforts?, *Health Affairs, 23*(2), 103-115.

6. Blendon, R. J., DesRoches, C. M., & Brodie, M. (2002) Views of practicing physicians and the public on medical errors. *New England Journal of Medicine, 347,* 1933-1940.

7. Posting to the National Patient Safety Foundation, *Patientsafety-L@listserv.npsf.org*, November 10, 2005.

8. Devers, K. J., Pham, H. H., & Liu, G. (2004). What is driving hospitals' patient-safety efforts?, *Health Affairs, 23*(2), 103-115.

9. Findings based in *Industrial Safety & Hygiene News'* "White Paper Study" (published by BNP Media), a mail survey of 511 *ISHN* subscribers conducted in August, 2004.

10. Findings based in *Industrial Safety & Hygiene News'* "White Paper Study" (published by BNP Media), a mail survey of 607 *ISHN* subscribers conducted in August, 2002.

11. Geller, E. S. (2005). *People-based safety: The source.* Virginia Beach, VA: Coastal Training Technologies Corp.

12. The common term is "near miss," but because of the literal meaning of a near miss, we prefer "near hit" or "close call."

13. The claim that 80-95% of injuries in general industry workplace are due in part to at-risk behavior is traced back to research by H.W. Heinrich, an assistant superintendent of the Engineering and Inspection Division of Travelers Insurance Company during the 1930s and 1940s. Heinrich reviewed supervisor accident reports and concluded 88% of all industrial accidents were primarily caused by unsafe acts. DuPont Safety Resources consultants say 96% of injuries and illnesses are caused by unsafe acts. Behavioral Science Technology (BST) has stated between 80% and 95% of all accidents are caused by unsafe behavior.

14. Pittet, D., Simon, A., Hugonnet, S., Pessoa-Silva, C. L., Sauvan, V., & Perneger, T. V. (2004). Hand hygiene among physicians: performance, beliefs, and perceptions. *Annals of Internal Medicine, 141*(1), 1-8.

15. Geller, E. S. (2002). *The participation factor: How to increase involvement in occupational safety.* Des Plaines, IL: American Society of Safety Engineers.

16. For more on the power of language see Hayakawa, S. I. (1978). *Language in thought and action* (Fourth Edition), New York: Harcourt Brace Jovanovich Publishers.

17. Latane, B., & Darley, J. M. (1970). *The unresponsive bystander: Why doesn't he help?* New York: Appleton-Century Crafts; Schroesder, D. A., Penner, L. A., Dovidio, J. F., & Piliavin, J. A. (1995). *The psychology of helping and altruism: Problems and puzzles.* New York: McGraw-Hill, Inc.

18. For more on assertiveness training see the audiotape series entitled "Assertiveness: The right choice" by National Press Publications, 1991 (PO Box 2949, Shawnee Mission, KS).

19. Lerner, M. S. (1980). *The belief in a just world: A fundamental delusion.* New York: Plenum Press.

20. Deming, W. E. (1986). *Out of the crisis.* Cambridge, MA: Massachusetts Institute of Technology, Center for Advanced Engineering Study; Deming, W.E. (1993). *The new economics for industry, government, education.* Cambridge, MA: Massachusetts Institute of Technology, Center for Advanced Engineering.

21. Bartlett, D. L., & Steele, J. B. (2006). *Critical condition: How health care in America became big business — and bad medicine.* New York: Broadway (originally published in 2004 by Doubleday).

22. ibid. p. 50.

23. ibid. p. 50.

24. Nelson, E. C., Batalden, P. B., Godfrey, M. M., Headrick, L., Huber, T. P., Mohr, J. J., & Wasson, J. H. (2003). Microsystems in health care: The essential building blocks of high performing systems. *The Joint Commission Journal of Quality Safety, 29*(11), 575-585.

25. "JCAHO proposes new patient safety goals," CCH Chicago Bureau, Dec. 8, 2005.

26. Gladwell, M. (2002). *The tipping point: How little things can make a big difference.* Boston: Back Bay Books (originally published in 2000 by Little, Brown and Company).

27. ibid. p. 221.

Chapter 2

1. Survey conducted by the American Association of Diabetes Educators was reported in the WebMD feature, *Beyond blood sugar: Testing A1c,* reviewed by Charlotte E. Grayson, MD, April, 2005.

2. Nightingale, F. (1969). *Notes on nursing.* New York: Dover Publications, Inc.

3. ibid. p. 45

4. ibid. pp. 48-49

5. ibid. p. 94

6. ibid. p. 125

7. For a review of the supportive research see Geller, E. S. (2001). *The psychology of safety handbook.* Boca Raton, FL: CRC Press. (Chapters 15 & 16).

8. Skinner, B. F. (1953). *Science and human behavior.* New York: Free Press; Skinner, B. F. (1974). *About behaviorism.* New York: Alfred A. Knopf.

9. Devers, K. J., Pham, H. H., & Liu, G. (2004). What is driving hospitals' patient-safety efforts? *Health Affairs, 23*(2), 103-115.

10. Entwistle, V. A., Mello, M. M., & Brennan, T. A. (2005). Advising patients about patient safety. *Journal on Quality and Patient Safety, 31*(9), 491.

11. Taylor, J. A., Brownstein, D., Christakis, D. A., Blackburn, S., Strandjord, T. P., Klein, E. J., & Shafii, J. (2004). Use of incident reports by physicians and nurses to document medical errors in pediatric patients. *Pediatrics, 114*(3), 729-735.

12. Cullen, D. J., Bates, D. W., Small, S. D., Cooper, J. B., Nemeskal, A. R., & Leape, L. L. (1995). The incident reporting system does not detect adverse drug event: A problem for quality improvement. *Joint Commission Journal on Quality Improvement, 21*, 541-548.

13. Flynn, E. A., Barker, K. N., Pepper, G. A., Bates, D. W., & Mikeal, R. L. (2002). Comparison of methods for detecting medication errors in 36 hospitals and skilled-nursing facilities. *American Journal of Health-System Pharmacy, 59*, 436-446.

14. Taylor, J. A., Brownstein, D., Christakis, D. A., Blackburn, S., Strandjord, T. P., Klein, E. J., & Shafii, J. (2004). Use of incident reports by physicians and nurses to document medical errors in pediatric patients. *Pediatrics, 114*(3), 729-735.

15. ibid.

16. ibid.

17. ibid.

18. ibid.

19. ibid.

20. ibid.

21. ibid.

22. ibid.

23. Norman, D. A. (1988). *The psychology of everyday things.* New York: Harper Collins Publishers.

24. Norman, D. A. (1988). *The psychology of everyday things.* New York: Harper Collins Publishers; Reason, J. T., & Mycieslka, K. (1982). *Absent minded? The psychology of mental lapses and everyday errors.* Englewood Cliffs, NJ: Prentice-Hall.

25. Heinrich, H. W. (1931). *Industrial accident prevention.* New York: McGraw-Hill.

26. Reported in Bird, Jr., F. E., & Davies, R. J. (1996). *Safety and the bottom line.* Loganville, GA: Institute Publishing, Inc.

27. Pittet, D., Simon, A., Hugonnet, S., Pessoa-Silva, C. L., Sauvan, V., & Perneger, T. V. (2004). Hand hygiene among physicians: Performance, beliefs, and perceptions. *Annals of Internal Medicine, 141*(1), 1-8.

28. ibid.

29. Private correspondence with author Dave Johnson, October, 2005. Nurse providing information requested anonymity.

30. Pittet, D., Simon, A., Hugonnet, S., Pessoa-Silva, C. L., Sauvan, V., & Perneger, T. V. (2004). Hand hygiene among physicians: Performance, beliefs, and perceptions. *Annals of Internal Medicine, 141*(1), 1-8.

31. ibid.

32. ibid.

33. ibid.

34. Nightingale, F. (1969). *Notes on nursing.* New York: Dover Publications, Inc.

35. Geller, E. S. (2001). *Psychology of safety handbook.* Boca Raton, FL: CRC Press

36. Pittet, D., Simon, A., Hugonnet, S., Pessoa-Silva, C. L., Sauvan, V., & Perneger, T. V. (2004). Hand hygiene among physicians: performance, beliefs, and perceptions. *Annals of Internal Medicine, 141*(1), 1-8.

37. Taylor, J. A., Brownstein, D., Christakis, D. A., Blackburn, S., Strandjord, T. P., Klein, E. J., & Shafii,

38. J. (2004). Use of incident reports by physicians and nurses to document medical errors in pediatric patients. *Pediatrics, 114*(3), 729 735.

39. *Medical errors: The scope of the problem.* Fact sheet, Publication No. AHRQ 00-P037. Agency for Healthcare Research and Quality, Rockville, MD.; *http://www.ahrq.gov/qual/errback.htm*

40. Centers for Disease Control and Prevention, National Center for Health Statistics, 2002 National Ambulatory Medical Care Survey.

41. U.S. Census Bureau, April 2005.

42. Centers for Disease Control and Prevention, National Center for Health Statistics, 2003 National Hospital Discharge Survey.

43. U.S. Census Bureau, April 2005.

44. Graber, M. (2005). Diagnostic errors in medicine. *Journal on Quality and Patient Safety, 31*(2), 112.

45. Lepper, M., & Greene, D. (1978) (Eds.). *The hidden cost of reward.* Hillsdale, NJ: Erlbaum.

46. Geller, E. S. (2001). *The psychology of safety handbook.* Boca Raton, FL: CRC Press.

47. Cialdini, R. B. (2001). *Influence: Science and practice* (Fourth Edition). New York: Harper Collin College Publishers; Geller, E. S. (2002). Social influence principles: Fueling participation in occupational safety. *Professional Safety, 47*(10), 25-31.

48. Cialdini, R. B., Cacioppo, J. T., Basset, R., & Miller, J. A. (1978). Low-ball procedure for producing compliance: Commitment then cost. *Journal of Applied Social Psychology, 15,* 492-500.

49. Freedman, J. L., & Fraser, S. C. (1966). Compliance without pressure: The foot-in-the-door technique. *Journal of Personality and Social Psychology, 4,* 195-203.

50. Berkowitz, L., & Daniels, L. R. (1963). Responsibility and dependency. *Journal of Abnormal and Social Psychology, 66,* 429-436.

51. Grote, D. (1995). *Discipline without punishment.* New York: American Management Association.

Chapter 3

1. Krisco, K. H. (1977). *Leadership and the art of conversation.* Rocklin, CA: Prima Publishing.

2. More information on the nondirective approach to interpersonal conversation is available in Rogers, C. R. (1961). *On becoming a person: A therapist's view of psychotherapy.* Boston, MA: Houghton Mifflin; and in Rogers, C. R. (1980). *A way of being.* Boston, MA: Houghton Mifflin.

3. John Drebinger provides more practical advice for effective safety communication in his book: Drebinger, Jr., J. W. (1998). *Master safety communication.* Galt, CA: Wulamoc Publishing.

4. James, W. (1890). *The principles of psychology.* New York: Holt.

5. Thorndike, E. L. (1911) *Animal intelligence: Experimental studies.* New York: Hofner; Thorndike, E. L. (1932). *Fundamentals of learning.* New York: Teachers College Press.

6. Case Study: Promoting high reliability surgery at Kaiser Permanente. Nov. 2004. The Commonwealth Fund. For further information see: DeFontes, J., & Surbida, S. (2004). Preoperative safety briefing project. *Permanente Journal, 8,* 21-27.

7. Tuckman, B. W. (1965). Developmental sequence in small groups. *Psychological Bulletin, 63,* 384-399.

8. Carnegie, D. (1936). *How to win friends and influence people* (Revised Edition). New York: Galahad Books.

9. Covey, S. R. (1989). *The seven habits of highly effective people.* New York: Simon & Schuster.

10. Gawande, A. (2002). *Complications.* New York: Picador.

11. Gardner, H. (1995). *Leading minds, an anatomy of leadership.* New York: Basic Books.

12. Gawande, A. (2002). *Complications.* New York: Picador.

13. 2004 Job Satisfaction Survey, conducted by the Society for Human Resource Management and CNNfn, the financial network of the CNN News.

14. Gardner, H. (1995). *Leading minds, an anatomy of leadership.* New York: Basic Books.

15. ibid. p. 289.

16. ibid. p. 286.

17. ibid. p. 291.

18. Entwistle, V. A., Mello, M. M., & Brennan, T. A. (2005). Advising patients about patient safety. *Journal on Quality and Patient Safety, 31*(9), 483-494.

19. Bandura, A. (1997). *Self-efficacy: The exercise of control.* New York: W. H. Freeman and Company; Geller, E. S. (2002). *The participation factor: How to increase involvement in occupational safety.* Des Plaines, IL: American Society of Safety Engineers.

20. Deci, E. L. (1975). *Intrinsic motivation.* New York: Plenum; Deci, E. L., & Ryan, R. M. (1985). *Intrinsic motivation and self-determination in human behavior.* New York: Plenum; Kohn, A. (1993). Punished by rewards: *The trouble with gold stars, incentive plans, A's, praise, and other bribes.* Boston: Houghton-Mifflin; Lepper, M. & Green, D. (1978) (Eds.). *The hidden cost of reward.* Hillsdale, NJ: Erlbaum.

Chapter 4

1. Taylor, J. A., Brownstein, D., Christakis, D. A., Blackburn, S., Strandjord, T. P., Klein, E. J., & Shafii, J. (2004). Use of incident reports by physicians and nurses to document medical errors in pediatric patients. *Pediatrics, 114*(3), 729-735.

2. Festinger, L. (1957). *A theory of cognitive dissonance.* Stanford, CA: Stanford University Press.

3. Iezzoni, L. I., (2005). *Discharged blindly.* Morbidity and mortality rounds on the web, Agency for Healthcare Research and Quality. *www.webmm.ahrq.gov.*

4. Theodorakis, Y. (2001). Self-talk in a basketball-shooting task. *Perceptual & Motor Skills, 92*(1), 309-315.

5. Anderson, O. (2005). *Science of sport: What to do when your brain imagines fatigue.* Posted on Running Research News. www.runnersweb.com.

6. Pittet, D., Simon, A., Hugonnet, S., Pessoa-Silva, C. L., Sauvan, V., & Perneger, T. V. (2004). Hand hygiene among physicians: Performance, beliefs, and perceptions. *Annals of Internal Medicine, 141*(1), 1-8.

7. Lindenaur, P. (2004). *Moved too soon.* Morbidity and mortality rounds on the web, Agency for Healthcare Research and Quality. *www.webmm.ahrq.gov.*

8. Watson, D. C., & Tharp, R. C. (1997). *Self-directed behavior: Self-modification for personal adjustment.* Seventh Edition. Pacific Grove, CA: Brooks/Cole Publishing.

9. Suinn, R. M. (1993). Imagery. In R. N. Singer, M. Murphey, & L. K. Tennent (Eds.), *Handbook on research in sport psychology,* 492-510. New York: Macmillan; Suinn, R. M. (1997). Mental practice in sport psychology: Where have we been, where do we go? *Clinical Psychology: Science and Practice, 4,* 189-207.

10. Rushall, B. (1988). *Self-efficacy and sports performance.* Posted on the web site *http://www-rohan.sdsu.edu/dept/coachsci/csa/vol14/rushall5.htm*

11. ibid.

12. Grainger, R. D. (1991). The use – and abuse—of negative thinking. *American Journal of Nursing, 91*(8), 13-14.

13. Bandura, A. (1997). *Self-efficacy: The exercise of control.* New York: W.H. Freeman and Company.

14. Bandura, A. (1997). The power of self-persuasion. *American Psychologist, 54,* 875-885; Seligman, M.E.P. (1991). *Learned optimism.* New York: Alfred A. Knopf.

15. Covellow, V. T., Sandman, P. M., & Slovic, P. (1991). Guidelines for communication information about chemical risk effectively and responsibly. In D. G. Mayo & R. D. Hollander (Eds.). *Acceptable evidence: Science and values in risk management* (pp. 66-90). New York: Oxford University Press.

16. Graber, M. (2005). Diagnostic errors in medicine. *Journal on Quality and Patient Safety, 31*(2), 114.

17. Blendon, R. J. *et al.* (2002). Views of practicing physicians and the public on medical errors. *New England Journal of Medicine, 347,* 1933-1940.

18. Skinner, B. F. (1953). *Science and human behavior.* New York: Free Press.

19. Graber, M. (2005). Diagnostic errors in medicine. *Journal on Quality and Patient Safety, 31*(2), 115.

20. ibid. p. 115.

21. Kruger, J., & Dunning, D. (1999). Unskilled and unaware of it: How difficulties in recognizing one's own incompetence lead to inflated self-assessments. *Journal of Personality and Social Psychology, 77*(6), 1121-1134.

22. ibid.

23. ibid.

24. Gawande, A. (2002). *Complications.* New York: Picador.

25. ibid.

26. Schyve, P. M. (2004). An interview with Lucian Leape. *The Joint Commission Journal on Quality and Safety, 31*(12).

27. Private correspondence with coauthor Dave Johnson, October, 2005. Physician requested anonymity.

28. Posting on the National Patient Safety Foundation listserv, Wed. Oct. 12, 2005.

29. Wachter, R. M. (2005). *Low on the totem pole*. Morbidity and mortality rounds on the web, Agency for Healthcare Research and Quality. www.webmm.ahrq.gov.

30. Langer, E. J. (1998). *Mindfulness*. Reading, MA: Perseus Books.

31. Gawande, A. (2002). *Complications*. New York: Picador.

32. Graber, M. (2005). Diagnostic errors in medicine. *Journal on Quality and Patient Safety, 31*(2), 113.

33. ibid. p. 113.

34. ibid. p. 113.

35. Private correspondence with coauthor Dave Johnson, October, 2005. Physician requested anonymity.

36. Graber, M. (2005). Diagnostic errors in medicine. *Journal on Quality and Patient Safety, 31*(2), 115.

37. Bartlett, D. L., & Steele, J. B. (2006). *Critical condition: How health care in America became big business — and bad medicine*. New York: Broadway (originally published in 2004 by Doubleday).

38. Aiken, L., Clarke, S., Sloane, D., Sochalski, J., & Silber, J. (2002). Hospital nurse staffing and patient mortality, nurse burnout, and job dissatisfaction. *Journal of the American Medical Association, 346*(22), 1715-1722.

39. Rogers, A. E., Hwang, W. T., Scott, L. D., Aiken, L. H., & Dinges, D. F. (2004). The working hours of hospital staff nurses and patient safety. *Health Affairs, (23)*4, 202-212.

40. ibid.

41. Draft Candidate 2007 National Patient Safety Goals, Requirements and Implementation Expections. Hospital and Critical Access Hospital Programs. P.9. Posted at: www.jcaho.org/.../critical+access+hospitals/ standards/draft+standards/07_npsg_hap_cah.pdf –

42. Wachter, R. M. (2005). *Low on the totem pole*. Morbidity and mortality rounds on the web, Agency for Healthcare Research and Quality. www.webmm.ahrq.gov.

43. Kruger, J., & Dunning, D. (1999). Unskilled and unaware of it: How difficulties in recognizing one's own incompetence lead to inflated self-assessments. *Journal of Personality and Social Pyschology, (77)*6, 1121-1134.

44. Langer, E. J. (1998). *Mindfulness*. Reading, MA: Perseus Books

45. Mager, R., & Pipe, P. (1997). *Analyzing performance problems or you really oughta wanna* (Third Edition). Atlanta, GA: Center for Effective Performance.

46. Atkinson, J. W. (1964). An introduction to motivation. Princeton, NJ: Van Nostand; McCelland, D. C. (1961). *The achieving society*. Princeton, NJ: Van Nostrand.

47. Geller, E. S. (2001). *Beyond safety accountability* (Second Edition). Rockville, MD: Government Institutes; Wiegand, D. M., & Geller, E. S. (2005). Connecting positive psychology and organizational behavior management: Achievement motivation and the power of positive reinforcement. *Journal of Organizational Behavior Management, 24*(1/2), 3-25.

Chapter 5

1. Langer, E. (1989) *Mindfulness*. Reading, MA: Addison-Wesley

2. Iezzoni, L. I., (2005). *Discharged blindly*. Morbidity and mortality rounds on the web, Agency for Healthcare Research and Quality. ***www.webmm.ahrq.gov***.

3. Lindenaur, P. (2004). *Moved too soon.* Morbidity and mortality rounds on the web, Agency for Healthcare Research and Quality. *www.webmm.ahrq.gov.*

4. *Color-coded wristbands create unnecessary risk* (2005). National Patient Safety Foundation list-serv.

5. Smith. L. (2005). *One dose, fifty pills.* Morbidity and Mortality Rounds on the web, Agency for Healthcare Research and Quality. *www.webmm.ahrq.gov.*

6. Ibid.

7. Johnston, W., & Dark, V. (1986). Selective attention. *Annual Review of Psychology, 37,* 43-75; Mack, A., & Rock, I. (1998). *Inattentional blindness.* Cambridge, MA: MIT Press.

8. Graber, M. (2004). *Crushing chest pain: A missed opportunity.* Morbidity and Mortality Rounds on the web, Agency for Healthcare Research and Quality. *www.webmm.ahrq.gov.*

9. Berkowitz, L., & Daniels, L. R. (1964). Affecting the salience of the social responsibility norm: Effect of past help on the responses to dependency relationships. *Journal of Abnormal and Social Psychology, 68,* 275-281.

10. Lerner, M. S. (1980). *The belief in a just world: A fundamental delusion.* New York: Plenium Press.

11. For a more extensive discussion of these distortions of risk perception, see Mayo, D. G., & Hollander, R. D. (1991) (EDS). *Deceptible evidence: Science and values in risk management.* New York: Oxford University Press.

12. Goodwin, C. J. (1998). *Research in psychology* (Second Edition). New York: John Wiley & Sons, Inc.

13. More details regarding the root-cause myth are given in Geller, E. S. (2004). Assessing SH&E Research: Key principles and practical strategies improve understanding. *Professional Safety, 49*(9), 22-29.

14. Krause, T. R. (2002). Predicting safety success: Examine these nine factors. *Industrial Safety & Hygiene News, 36*(3), 52-53.

15. Cialdini, R. B. (2001). *Influence: Science and practice* (Fourth Edition). New York: Harper Collin College Publishers; Geller, E. S. (2002). Social influence principles: Fueling participation in occupational safety. *Professional Safety, 47*(10), 25-31.

16. Langer, E. J. (1989). *Mindfulness.* Reading, MA: Perseus Books.

17. Findings based on *Industrial Safety & Hygiene News'* "White Paper Study" (published by BNP Media), a mail survey of 494 *ISHN* subscribers conducted in August, 2003.

18. Private correspondence with coauthor Dave Johnson, December, 2005.

19. Petersen, D. (2000). Safety management 2000: Our strengths and weaknesses. *Professional Safety, 1,* 16-19.

20. ibid.

21. Wachter, R., M., & Shojania, K. G. (2004). *Internal bleeding: The truth behind America's terrifying epidemic of medical mistakes.* New York: Rugged Land. p.119.

22. Peltzman, S. (1975). The effects of automobile safety regulation. *Journal of Political Economics, 83,* 677-725; Adams, J. (1995). *Risk.* London: UCL Press; Wilde, G. J. S. (1994). *Target risk* (p. 228). Toronto, Ontario, Canada: PDE Publications.

23. University of Pennsylvania Medical Center. Press release posted at: *http://www.sci-encedaily.com/releases/2005/03/050309131334.htm.*

24. Patterson, E. S., Cook, R. I., & Render, M. L. (2002). Improving patient safety by identifying side effects from introducing bar coding in medication administration. *Journal of the American Medical Informatics Association. 9*(5), 540-553.

25. ibid.

26. ibid.

27. ibid.

28. ibid.

29. Deming, W. E. (1991, May). *Quality productivity and competitive position.* Four-day workshop presented in Cincinnati, Ohio, by Quality Enhancement Seminars, Inc.

30. Geller, E. S., Winett, R. A., & Everett, P. B. (1982). *Preserving the environment. New strategies for behavior change.* New York: Pergamon Press; Kazdin, A. E., & Wilson, G. T. (1978). *Evaluation of behavior therapy: Issues, evidence, and research strategies.* Cambridge, MA: Ballinger; Peterson, D. (1989). *Safe behavior reinforcement.* New York: Aloray, Inc.

31. Tillman, R., & Kirkpatrick, C. A. (1972). *Promotion: Persuasive communication in marketing.* Homewood, IL: Richard D. Irwin, Inc.

32. Van Houten, R., & Nau, P. A. (1983). Feedback interventions and driving speed: A parametric and comparative analysis. *Journal of Applied Behavior Analysis*, 16, 253-281.

33. Gawande, A. (2002). *Complications.* New York: Picador.

34. ibid.

35. Mack, A., & Rock, I. (1998). *Inattentional blindness.* Cambridge, MA: MIT Press.

Chapter 6

1. Geller, E.S. (1998). *Beyond safety accountability: How to increase personal responsibility.* Neenah, WI: J.J. Keller & Associates, Inc.

2. O'Neill, P. Speech delivered at the Workplace Safety Summit, Georgetown University, Washington, D.C., March 30, 2001.

3. Ibid.

4. Collins, J (2001). *Good to great.* New York: HarperCollins Publishers, Inc.

5. Rees, F. (1997). *Teamwork from start to finish.* San Francisco: Jossey-Boss, Inc.

6. Private correspondence with author Dave Johnson, October, 2005. Anonymity requested.

7. Creating top-of-mind-awareness. Byrd, R., & Nelson, R. (2005). Posted on the web site www.attractcustomers.com. Fast Forward Marketing & Public Relations.

8. ibid.

9. Private correspondence with author Dave Johnson, October, 2005. Anonymity requested.

10. Towers Perrin survey: Enhancing corporate credibility: Is it time to take the spin out of employee communications? Conducted by Harris Interactive in mid-year 2003. An online survey of 1,000 working Americans.

11. Gallup study: Feeling good matters in the workplace. Conducted by The Gallup Organization, October 2000–May 2005. About 1,000 employed adults aged 18 and older were interviewed by telephone.

12. The Conference Board study: U.S. job satisfaction keeps falling. Conducted by TNS. Report based on a representative sample of 5,000 U.S. Households, and also information collected independently by TNS. Findings released by The Conference Board February, 2005.

13. ibid.

14. Towers Perrin survey: Enhancing corporate credibility: Is it time to take the spin out of employee communications? Conducted by Harris Interactive in mid-year 2003. An online survey of 1,000 working Americans.

15. Crawford. C. (2003). You must create top of mind awareness. *Limitless Marketing Ezine.* Crawford Marketing Consultants, www.williecrawford.com.

16. Abraham, M. (2001). Top of mind awareness in industrial markets: Why you need to get and keep it! Posted on sticky-marketing.net, *www.sticky-marketing.net.*

17. Ken Blanchard calls this "situational leadership" as introduced in Blanchard, K. P., Zigami, P., & Zigarini, D. (1985). *Leadership and the one-minute manager.* New York: William Morrow and Company, Inc.

18. Geller, E. S. (1999 March). Building momentum for safety. *Industrial Safety & Hygiene News,* 33(3), pp.16,18 ; Mace, F. C., Lalli, J. S., Shea, M. C., & Nevin, J. A. (1992) Behavior momentum in college basketball. *Journal of Applied Behavior Analysis,* 25, 657-667.

19. Gallup study: Feeling good matters in the workplace. Conducted by The Gallup Organization, October 2000-May 2005. About 1,000 employed adults aged 18 and older were interviewed by telephone.

20. The Conference Board study: U.S. job satisfaction keeps falling. Conducted by TNS. Report based on a representative sample of 5,000 U.S. Households, and also information collected independently by TNS. Findings released by The Conference Board February, 2005.

21. Berkowitz, L., & Daniels, L. R. (1964). Affecting the salience of the social responsibility norm: Effect of past help on the responses to dependency relationships. *Journal of Abnormal and Social Psychology,* 68, 275-281.

22. For more on the social influence principles see Geller, E. S. (2002). Social influence principles: Fueling participation in occupational safety. *Professional Safety,* 47(10), 25–31.

Index

About the Authors

E. Scott Geller, Ph.D. is a Senior Partner of Safety Performance Solutions, Inc. – a leading-edge organization specializing in behavior-based safety training and consulting. Dr. Geller and his partners at Safety Performance Solutions (SPS) have helped companies across the country and around the world address the human dynamics of occupational safety through flexible research-founded principles and industry-proven tools. In addition, for almost four decades, Professor E. Scott Geller has taught and conducted research as a faculty member in the Department of Psychology at Virginia Polytechnic Institute and State University, better known as Virginia Tech. In this capacity, he has been the principal investigator on 80 research grants and has authored more 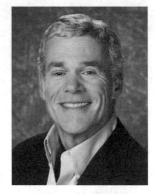 than 350 research articles and over 75 books or chapters addressing the development and evaluation of behavior-change interventions to improve quality of life. Dr. Geller is an Alumni Distinguished Professor, and a Fellow of the American Psychological Association, the Association of Psychological Science, and the World Academy of Productivity and Quality Sciences.

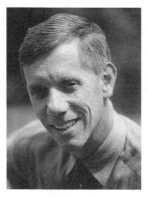 *Dave Johnson* is a journalist, editor and researcher with more than 25 years of experience reporting on organizational safety issues. His over 500 magazine feature articles have covered topics including world-class organizational safety cultures, management systems, senior leadership for safety, behavioral safety, close calls, complacency, selling safety to executives, safety coaching and teamwork, perception surveys, risk assessment, techno stress, performance metrics, and gaining employee buy-in. Johnson has also reported on safety culture improvement efforts at NASA, the Los Alamos Testing Laboratory, and Fortune 500 corporations. In 1995, he edited Dr. E. Scott Geller's book, *The Psychology of Safety*. Dave has presented research findings and issues and trends updates at scores of safety society and association conferences across the United States. He lives outside Philadelphia, Pennsylvania.